8/30/75

To Ray +

Its great
visiting with you.
God Love You +
Bless You Always,

John Burak

THERE GOES MY ACHING BACK

THERE GOES MY ACHING BACK

John Burak, B. S., R. P. T.
Registered Physical Therapist
Member of American Physical Therapy Association

Foreword by

DONALD D. SMITH, M.D.
American Board Orthopedic Surgery
Fellow American College of Surgeons
American Academy, Orthopedic Surgery

An Exposition-Banner Book

Exposition Press Hicksville, New York

First Edition

Inquiries should be addressed to Exposition Press, Inc.,
900 South Oyster Bay Road, Hicksville, N.Y. 11801

Library of Congress Catalog Card Number: 74-21437

ISBN 0-682-48134-3

Printed in the United States of America

To all my immediate family,
especially to my parents
who, as young adults,
came to this country from Czechoslovakia
and always expected me
to do my best in all things.

CONTENTS

FOREWORD

I have used this type of program with Mr. Burak treating the majority of my back patients over the last nineteen years. I have found that this method particularly emphasizing the use of the abdominal muscles has been quite effective as long as the patient understands the program and understands how to apply it to the various activities that he carries out during the day.

From my own personal experience, I know that it works since I have had some back trouble. I also have had patients with back problems, for many years, that have improved a great deal or even had their pain subside under this program.

Donald D. Smith, M.D.
American Board Orthopedic Surgery
Fellow American College of Surgeons
American Academy, Orthopedic Surgery

PREFACE

The need for changing the present course of treatment and prevention of low back pain is much overdue.

According to recent statistics, eight million people injure their backs annually. Add to this the number of chronic back patients from the past years and the number becomes staggering and increasing each year.

Outside of improved methods of diagnosing and surgery, conservative treatment including bed rest, traction, heat, ultrasound, exercise, bracing, muscle relaxants, and pain pills is aimed at treating and relieving symptoms rather than causes. Consequently, the results are most questionable and the medical costs are astronomical.

Most pamphlets teaching people to lift with their legs and keep their backs straight are actually teaching people how to injure their backs.

Back pain is not only a medical and economical problem, but it is also a serious social, vocational, and psychological problem.

A man's greatest asset as the head of a household is his ability to produce and provide. When this ability to work as a laborer, electrician, plumber, or logger is threatened, he is confronted with a serious problem. In many cases he goes on as long as he can, enduring his pain and doing his job, or he changes to a job that he is able to do. Otherwise, he becomes unemployed and becomes a drain on our economy.

A man who is unproductive and idle, with constant pain, develops further problems. He is unable to attend social functions because he can't sit for very long at one time; he can't drive or ride in a car for any length of time; he can't sleep and rest properly and, therefore, becomes irritable and sensitive; he worries about his future—that he can't maintain his standard of living; he becomes ashamed that he can't "keep up with the Joneses." These can become serious social problems. Psychological problems develop within his family. He is unable to participate in family activities. He is unable to perform his sexual activities, and, therefore, creates a problem between himself and his wife. As time goes on, many problems become exaggerated; such a man becomes a good candidate for excessive drinking and begins to lose his spirit. Would you like to be in such a predicament? There are many such men, and they are not getting much help because they have no temperature, their X rays look normal, and they don't look sick.

A housewife with a painful back is not confronted with the important task of providing for her family, as long as her husband is productive; however, she, too, has many serious problems which can develop to great proportions. She, too, will become idle and handicapped physically. She will be unable to keep her house clean, make the beds, stand by a stove and do the cooking, pick up her children, and show love and affection for her family that she so much wants to. What problems will she develop? She will prefer to stay home rather than go along with her husband to social affairs such as the theater, ball games, and dances; the fun stops. She can't sleep, can't enjoy making love to her husband (what starts going on in his mind?). She becomes irritable, self-centered, sensitive; she's constantly yelling at her children; they don't want to be at home any more than they have to. The entire family is affected, which can lead to the most serious problem of all—the breaking up of the home.

As you can now understand, back pain can be a very serious problem, and to many people it is. That is why I decided to write this book. I feel that I have a new approach which is sound, simple, complete, and can be taught to most people.

I propose to prove that using the abdominal muscles properly is the most effective means of stopping back pain, strengthening the back, and preventing back injuries. I also intend to prove the typical belief that you must "Keep your back straight and use your legs in lifting to keep from injuring your back" is a fallacy.

I want to thank all the medical doctors in the Pendleton, Oregon area, and especially Dr. Donald D. Smith, orthopedic surgeon, who through the past nineteen years allowed me to decide the course of therapeutic exercise and approach to treating his back injured patients. My basic philosophy of treatment is the same today as it was nineteen years ago. The results of this type of treatment are just as dramatic today as they were fifteen years ago.

Finally, I want to thank Pat Murphy, who acted as the model for the photo illustrating, and Mrs. Dorothy Baskins, a faculty member at Blue Mountain Community College, who edited and typed my manuscript, and was a pleasure to work with.

THERE GOES MY ACHING BACK

Chapter I

CAUSE OF BACK PAIN

Back pain can come from many causes, such as a sudden injury, arthritis, poor posture, psychosomatic conditions, congenital malformations, cancer, kidney disease, multiple sclerosis, and many other diseases. Most medical doctors, with today's wonderful diagnostic means, are able to diagnose even the most serious causes of back pain. Because of the great variety of possible reasons for pain in one's back, one should go only to a medical doctor for diagnosis and treatment.

The most common cause is low back strain or sprain. A strain is usually defined as an injury to a muscle resulting from tension caused by overuse or misuse. A sprain is a sudden or violent wrenching of a joint, causing ligaments to stretch or rupture. In many cases, both are present. These conditions or injuries can be mild, moderate, or severe, with symptoms ranging from mild aching to severe pain in the back, and radiating into the lower extremities. In many people, the condition is recent acute and severe; in others, it is severe or mild and chronic, extending over a period of months and years. Many people have had chronic back pain since childhood.

What actually occurs to the low back when we say it is sprained? Usually, when we lift something heavy or something lighter suddenly, we arch our back too far backwards, stretching the muscles and ligaments that hold the last movable joints together in our low back. The result is similar to spraining an ankle.

If a person is swaybacked, he may, over a period of years, gradually accomplish the same injury at a slower pace. With the overstretching of these tissues that hold these lower spinal joints together, the result is excessive and abnormal motion in the low back. Accompanying this is irritation to tissue, which causes inflammation and swelling along with muscle spasm. The spasm occurs primarily to fixate the joint that is injured, so that further injury does not occur. This is nature's way of causing severe pain with any movement that may aggravate the condition. Severe symptoms, such as I have mentioned, occur in an acute back sprain, which is usually brought on by sudden injury. These symptoms can be similar, but mild, in a chronic back sprain caused by poor posture. Therefore, the cause of pain during movement results from the instability of the injured joint and increased pressure on the injured tissue around the joint. It is just too weak to maintain its normal position during movement. The swelling and acuteness of the condition aggravates the situation.

Chapter II

PRINCIPLES OF TREATMENT

TREATMENT AND PREVENTION

What I propose to do in this book is to explain and indicate how the use of the abdominal muscles is the most important and effective method in treating and preventing low back strain and sprain.

As mentioned earlier, in a low back sprain or strain the injury is to the supporting tissue around a low back joint, most commonly the last movable joint of the spine. The most common cause of the injury is a sudden extension of the back as in lifting, or a gradual, chronic swayback.

The best position for any joint to heal is when it is in a neutral or straight position. For example, a sprained ankle is most comfortable when it is in a straight alignment, since in this position there is the least amount of stress on the supportive tissue that is injured. The same applies with the low back.

In order for any joint to heal, you must place it in the best possible position and keep it in this position for the necessary period of time, allowing nature to heal the injured tissue. During this period of time, all irritation and strain must be eliminated or kept at a minimum. Since it is almost impossible to tell to what degree the joint has been weakened and the tissue injured, we must eliminate all stress, strain, and irritation. This must be done to obtain the most rapid healing.

Since the injury is caused by extending the back with the strong back muscles, any similar movement causes pain, irritation, and aggravation of the initial injury. By contracting or tightening the abdominal muscles, movement is in the opposite direction to the injury, and when the abdominals are completely contracted the low back is locked in the most favorable position to heal. The joint is in the most stable position and the patient will be pain-free. It has been my experience that if a patient keeps his low back in this position by the use of his abdominal muscles, he is able to perform all activities without pain.

The abdominal muscles act as a brace. In fact, there is no brace made that can compete with your abdominal muscles. The abdominal muscles prevent all movement in the low back. If there is no movement, there is no irritation—therefore, no pain. If there is no movement and no irritation, nature has the maximum opportunity to heal.

The amount of force used by the abdominals is proportional to the activity performed. Standing requires a small amount of abdominal force to prevent movement and maintain position. To get up from a chair requires more force. To lift a heavy weight requires maximum abdominal force to prevent motion and maintain stability. You must remember that any movement in an acute back sprain causes pain. This must be prevented.

If a person with low back pain can be taught how to prevent irritation and strain, he will cure himself. If a person uses his abdominals properly, he will never injure his back.

FUNCTIONAL TRAINING—ACTIVITIES OF DAILY LIVING

Man is basically lazy and functions with the least amount of energy possible. This, unfortunately, is the main cause of back trouble. If you were to tear down a house and you had a choice of using a crow bar or a hammer, you would naturally pick up the crow bar because of the tremendous leverage and the amount of energy it would save you. The same applies to a man or woman using his or her body. Why should he use the muscles of his legs, arms, and abdominals when he can, with much less effort, use the large lever of the entire spine?

Activities of daily living include working while standing, getting up and down from a chair, toilet, car seat, or bed, picking up objects from the floor, getting objects from low shelves, shopping in a supermarket, making a bed, working in a garden, working for a living, playing sports, reaching, twisting, and all the other activities of daily living that you can think of.

Practically all people performing their activities of daily living extend their backs in everything they do, as I will point out later on. Consequently, over a period of years their low back becomes weak and susceptible to injury. After they are injured they continue to use their backs in the same manner. Constantly, they are irritating themselves; treatment is prolonged if the injury is mild, and many times treatment is futile if the injury is severe. In many cases recurrent back trouble is common.

The most difficult problem I have in the treatment of patients is motivating them to use their abdominal muscles. To all people it is unnatural, as I mentioned earlier, and they are looking for some magic cure from someone which takes no effort on their part.

The success of this treatment is motivating people to use their abdominal muscles during all activities of daily living—twenty-four hours a day. I have come to the conclusion that no one can do as much for a low back strain as the person who can treat himself twenty-four hours a day.

I will now discuss the basic movements of the body that are used in all activities of living and working. I will show you how these activities can be performed without movement or strain in the lower spine by using the abdominal muscles properly.

CONTRACTING ABDOMINAL MUSCLES (figure 1)

What do I mean by contracting the abdominal muscles? If you ask people to tighten or contract their abdominal muscles, nine out of ten people will suck in their tummy and lift up their chest. While they are doing this they also are inhaling air. When you inhale it is impossible to use your abdominal muscles. All the sucking in is being done by the contraction of the diaphragm.

The abdominal muscles extend from the front of the rib cage to the pelvis. When they contract they bring the rib cage down towards your pubis, pelvis, or hips, and round your back. They are used strongly in forced expiration when breathing. This can be especially noticed when you blow up a balloon or when you cough. Most commonly the abdominals are used to do a "sit up" exercise.

When the abdominals are completely contracted the low back is completely flexed or flattened out. The upper back is rounded and no more movement is possible as long as the contraction is maintained; the abdomen is very firm.

RESTING

While you are resting, the important factor is that the injured joint or tissue is at complete rest. The most favorable position for any joint is the normal anatomical or neutral position. In most cases it is when the joint is straight.

While resting on your back (figure 2), pillows should be placed under your knees. The pillows will flex your hips and knees causing your pelvis to tilt back toward the bed, helping to flatten your low back and remove all the strain from your injured joint. If you are round shouldered or have a rounded back you should use a larger pillow under your head and shoulders. By doing this your rib cage will be tilted forward toward your pubis, helping to flatten the low back, especially the upper part of your low back.

While resting on your side (figure 3), the legs and knees should be flexed to about ninety degrees and a pillow placed between the knees and ankles. The hips being flexed tilts the pelvis backward and flattens the low back. The pillow between the legs keeps the top leg from pulling on the hip joint, which in turn prevents a pull on the pelvis, which in turn prevents a twist in the lumbar spine that would cause the strain and pain.

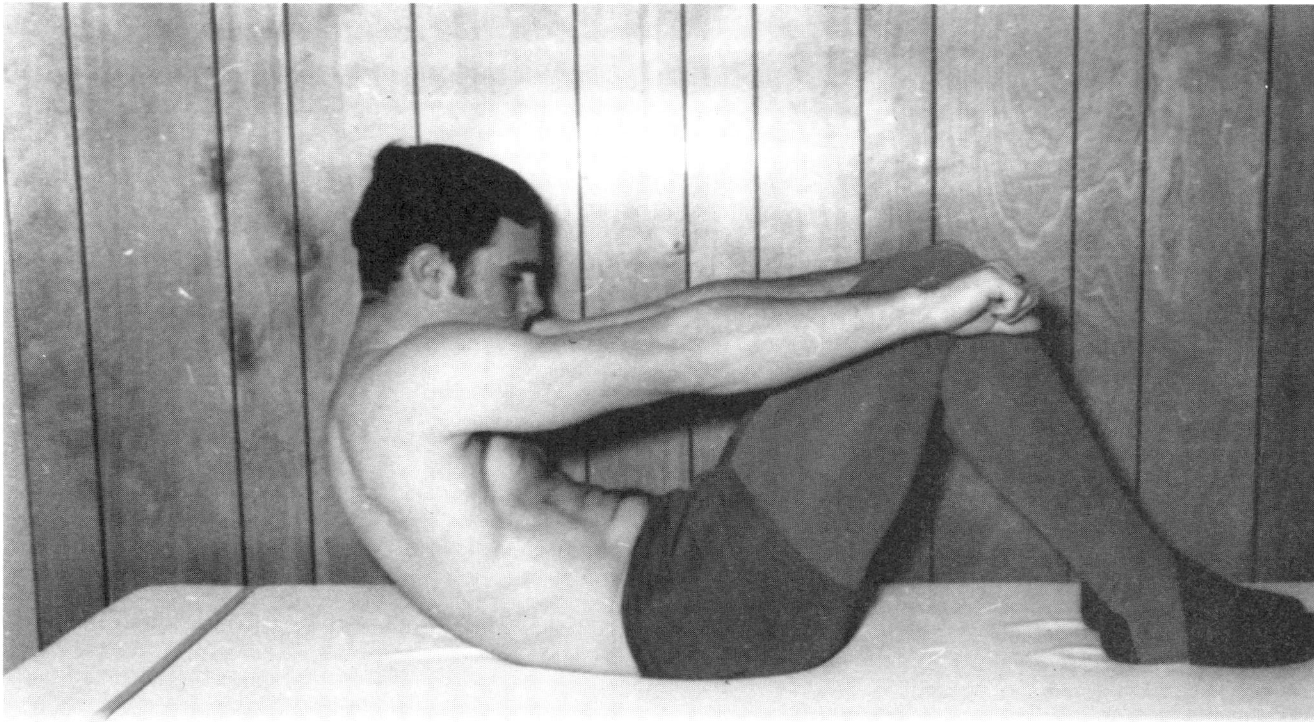

FIGURE 1 Contracting Abdominal Muscles

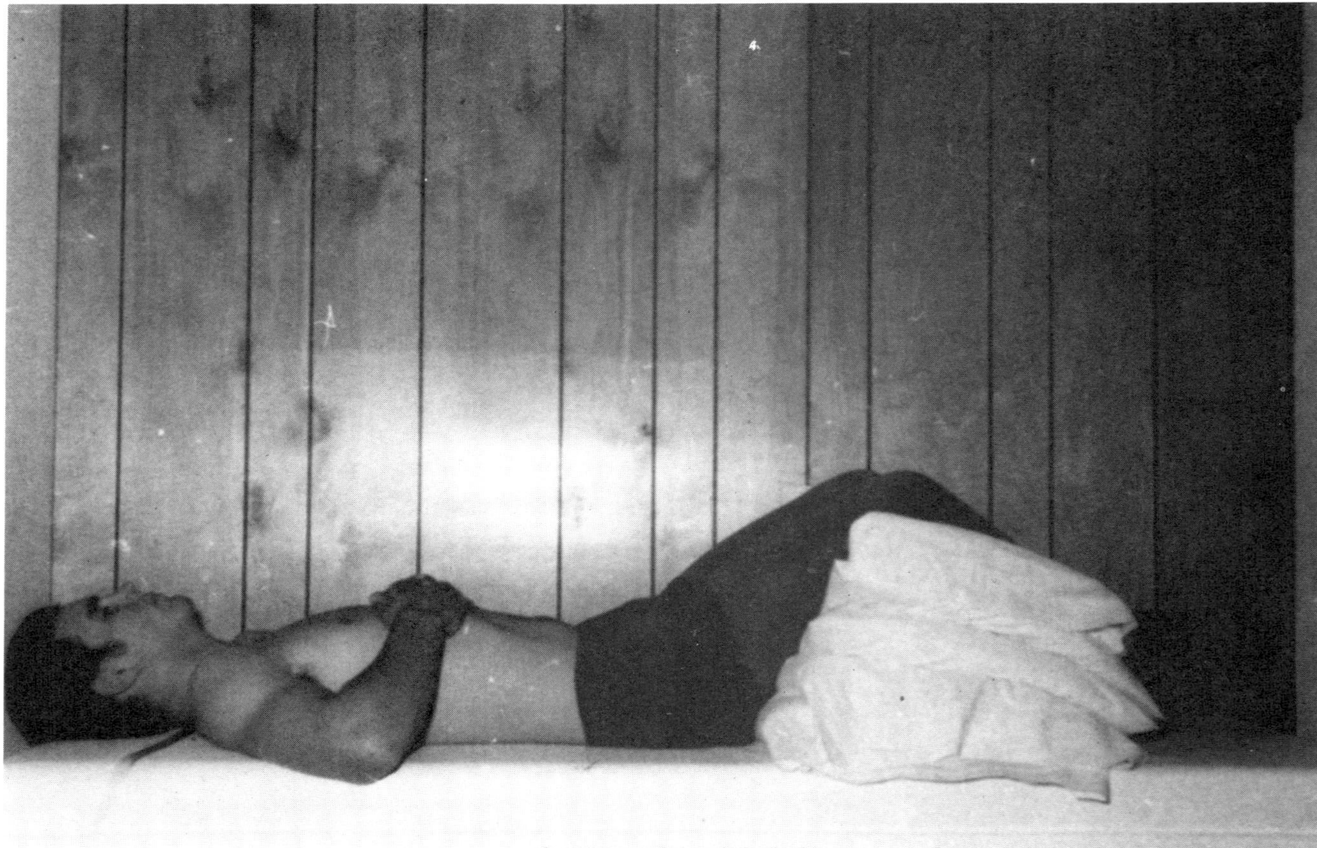

FIGURE 2 Resting on Your Back

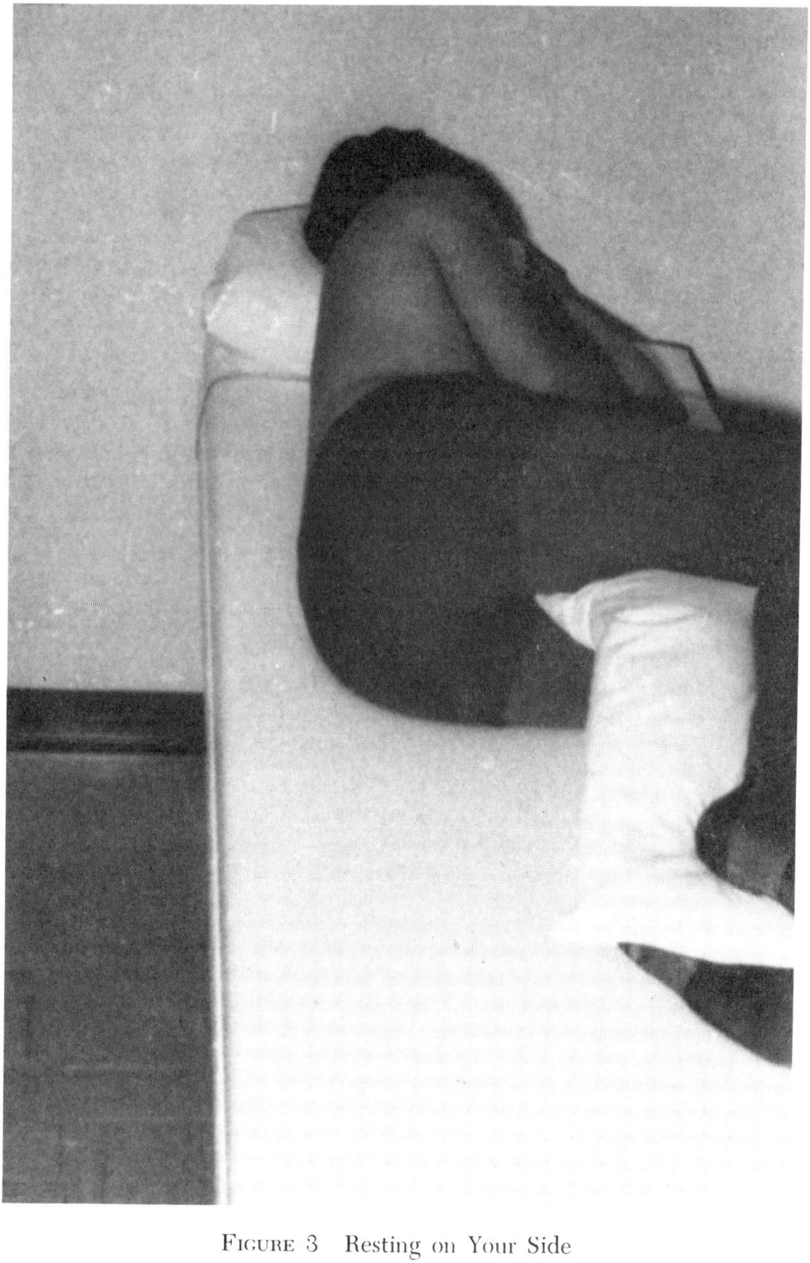

FIGURE 3 Resting on Your Side

Resting on your stomach (figure 4) should be discouraged since getting on and off your stomach is difficult to do without severe strain. However, if you must, you should have enough pillows under your abdomen to flatten your low back completely. If you are not comfortable, most likely you don't have enough pillows under you.

Resting in a standing position (figure 5) is difficult. This can be done by placing one foot on a chair or a box which will flatten the low back. However, dropping the hip on one side may still occur if you relax your abdominal muscles. Therefore, resting on both feet may be easier if you use your abdominals just enough to keep the back flat to give you a feeling of sitting on your legs.

Most people find resting in a sitting position (figure 6) most difficult, and most people with injured or painful backs find that sitting aggravates their condition.

When most people sit, they place their buttocks in the middle of the chair and then completely relax. By doing this all muscular support is taken away and the vertebrae of the low back are in a bowed out position. All the weight from the low back up is hanging on the low back. When the upper back is placed against the back rest and the muscles relaxed, the entire back then tends to slip forward on the pelvis that you are sitting on (figure 6b). This causes a forward shearing especially forceful at the last movable joint which involves the last lumbar vertebrae on the pelvis and sacrum. When one relaxes in the sitting position the weight of the body will move in the direction with the least amount of resistance, the same as water running down a hill. Consequently, the tissue that is the weakest would be irritated the most and cause strain and pain.

It is interesting to note that most people with back trouble will prefer to sit in a straight-backed hard chair. They get most comfort from this type of a chair because the injured joint and tissue are maintained in a more neutral position which lessens strain.

By placing your pelvis as far back into any seat as possible, you will keep your pelvis straight. If you sit on a hard straight-

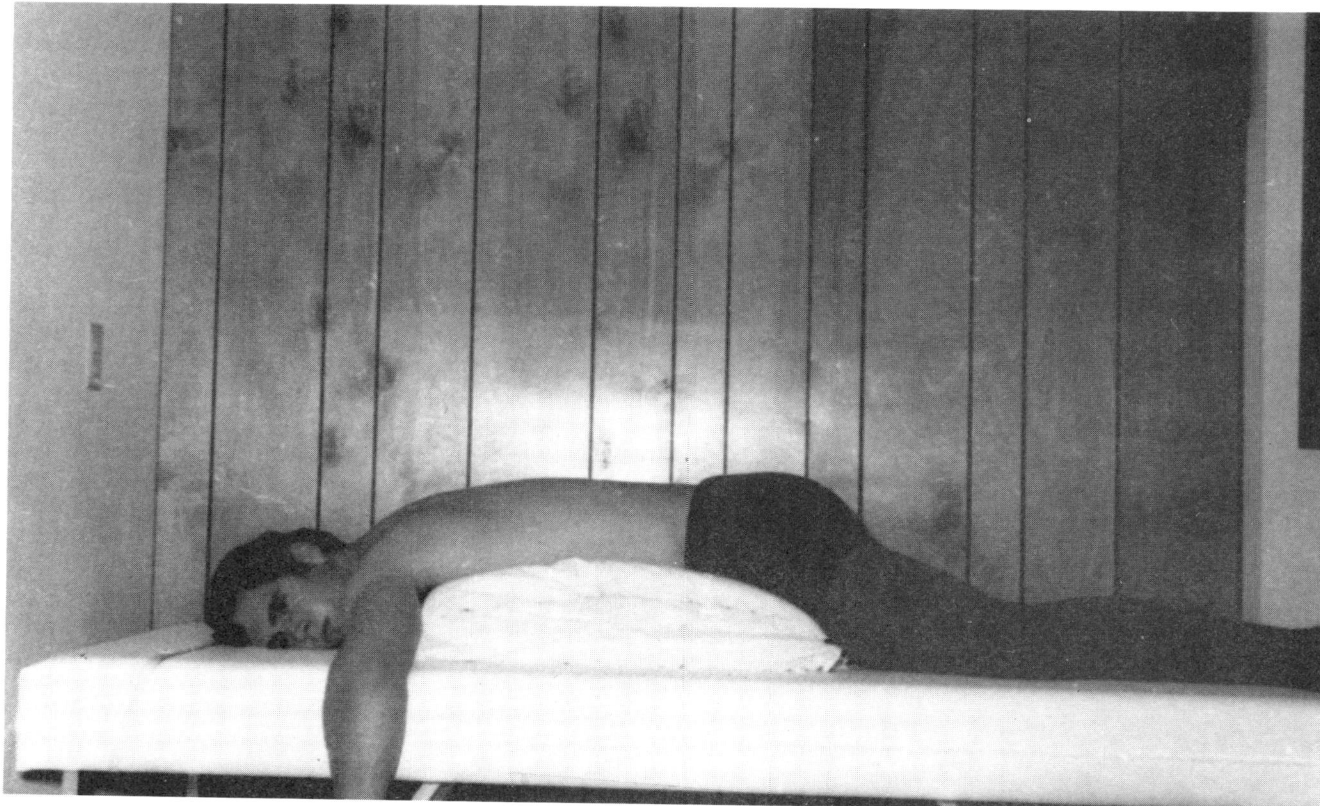

Figure 4 Resting on Stomach

FIGURE 5 Standing

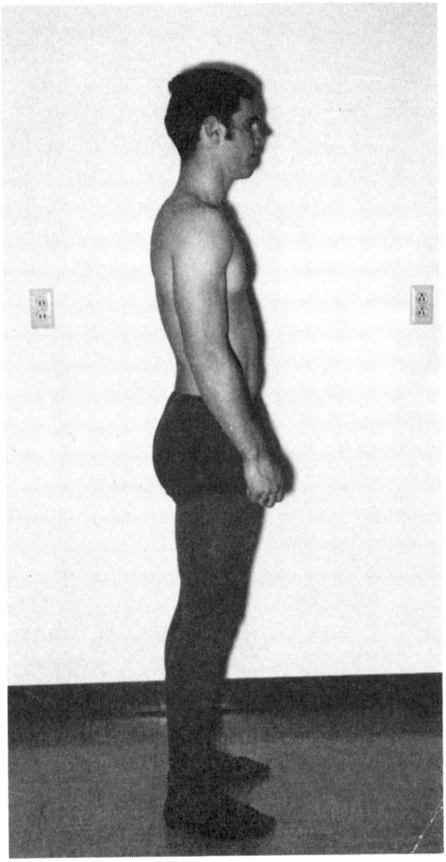

(Abdominals Relaxed)

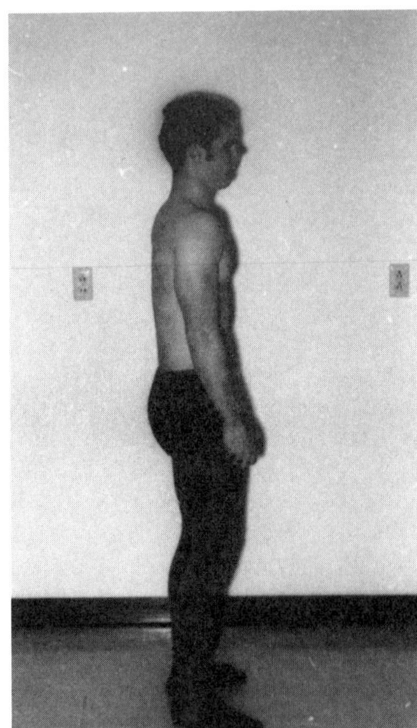

(Abdominals Contracted)

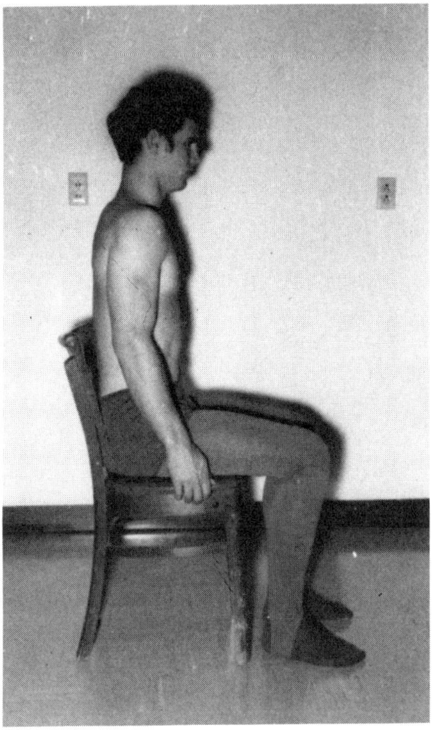

FIGURE 6 Proper Sitting

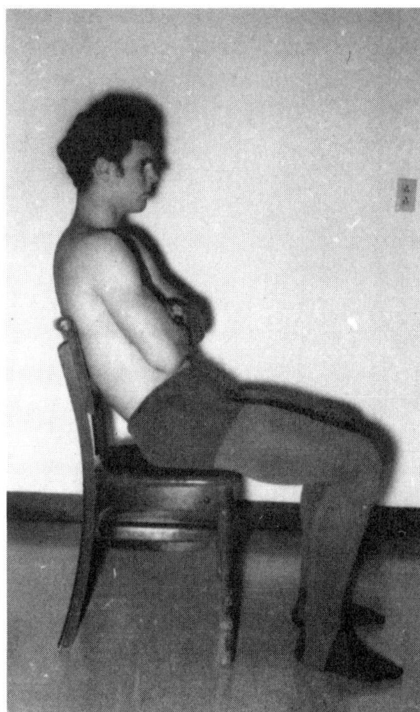

FIGURE 6b Improper Sitting

backed chair with the pelvis back against the straight-backed chair, your back cannot bow out; your body weight will keep your low back straight and the center of gravity will be going through the center or in front of your spine, preventing a shearing effect. If you are not sitting in a firm straight-backed chair, keep your back straight with your muscles. Do not relax, and you may be able to sit for much longer periods. You would be wiser to lie down in a proper position rather than relax in a poor sitting position.

Chapter III

BASIC MOVEMENTS OF THE BODY

BED ACTIVITIES

Almost all back patients have pain when they try to move in bed. Because the low back is the center of the body, all movements affect the low back. The pain is initiated by motion in the low back.

The most comfortable position in bed is when the patient is on his back with knees flexed and feet flat on the bed. This position can be maintained with many pillows under the knees or by rolling up the hospital bed. The knees should be as high as possible, giving the maximum relief by flattening the low back.

Moving the hips from one side of the bed to the other is usually very painful since most patients use their elbows and lift their hips and low back up off the bed to move over. The lifting of the hips and low back extends or arches the back and pain is initiated by movement of the injured joint.

To move from side to side in bed without pain (figure 7), first raise your head, shoulders, and arms up from the bed until the abdominal muscles are firm. Secondly, move your feet over to the side toward which you wish to go. Then, by using your feet, lift your hips up from the bed and then swing the hips. All motion takes place in the hip joints and there is no pain in the

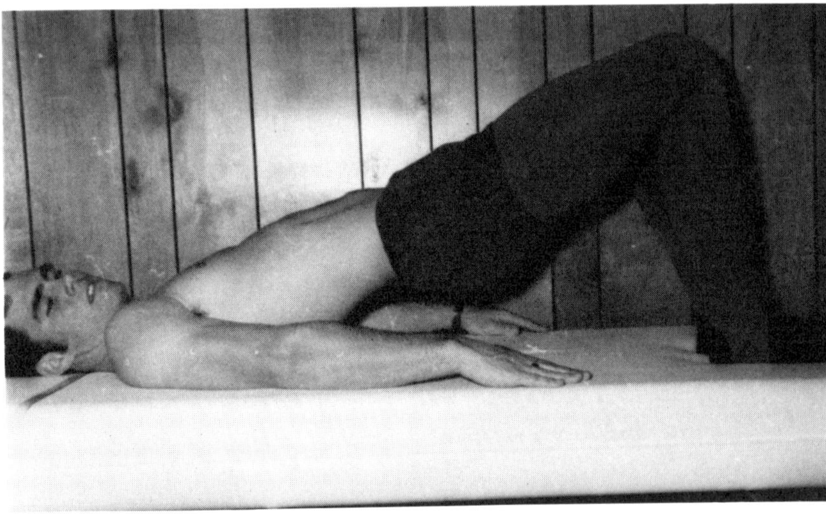

(Moving the Hips with Abdominals Relaxed)

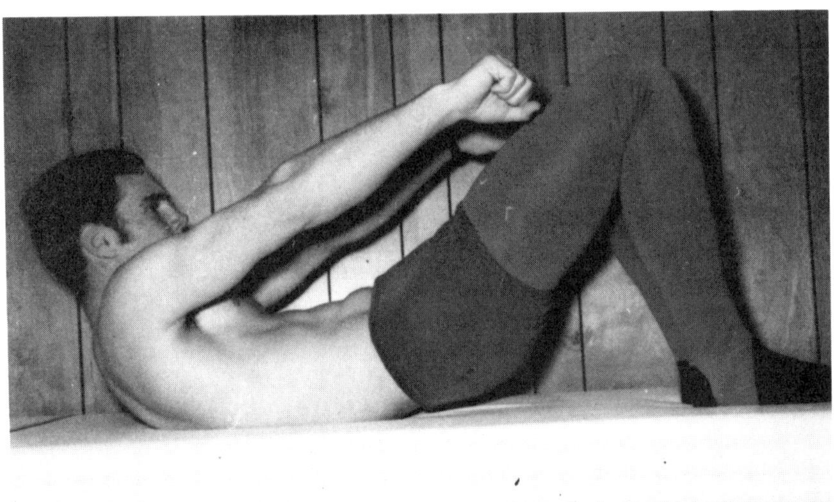

(Moving the Hips with Abdominals Contracted)

Figure 7 Moving Hips in Bed

low back. You must not use your elbows. To move the head and shoulders to the same side, you again raise the head, shoulders, and arms, and you side-bend with your lateral trunk muscles. Then, drop your head and shoulders in the same line as your hips and feet.

When you are lying on your back and you want to turn on your side (figure 8), raise the head, shoulders, and arms until your abdominals are firm. Then fall or roll the entire body on its side, all in one unit, just as a log rolls. With the abdominals firm, you will not experience pain since there is no movement or irritation in the low back. If you relax your muscles you will experience pain as soon as motion is allowed in the injured joint. Returning from the side-lying position to the back position the same principle is applied.

In moving from the head of the bed to the foot of the bed (figure 9), you must raise the head, shoulders, and arms until the abdominals are as firm as possible without pain. Then you place your hands on the bed behind the hips and push with your hands and feet, lifting up the buttocks, and swing your body toward your feet at the hips, knees, and shoulders. When moving toward the head of the bed, the same principle and procedure is followed, except that the feet are placed close to the buttocks and the hands toward the head of the bed. The trunk swings away from the feet and toward the hands. Pain will not be experienced since there is no movement or irritation. You may also go forward or down toward the foot of the bed, moving on your side, by first turning on your side and then moving, keeping the abdominals firm.

A patient should never be asked to lie on a bed pan unless the head of the bed is much higher than the hips, and his back is straight and pain-free while he is on the pan.

SITTING UP ON THE EDGE OF A BED

When moving from a back-lying position with the knees flexed to a sitting position on the edge of the bed (figure 10), you must

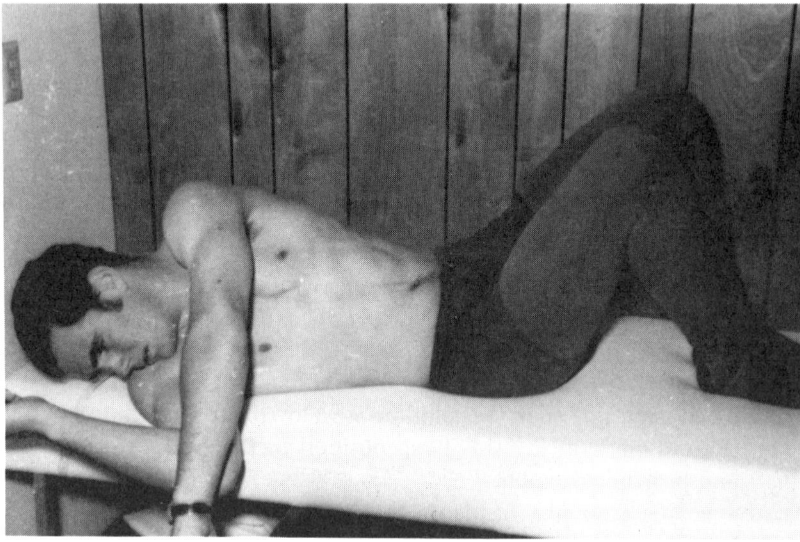

(Abdominals Relaxed)

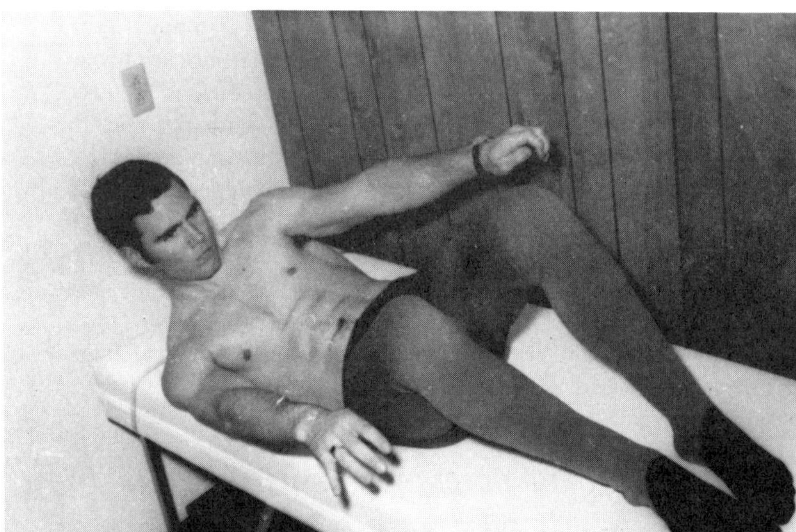

(Abdominals Contracted)

FIGURE 8 Turning in Bed

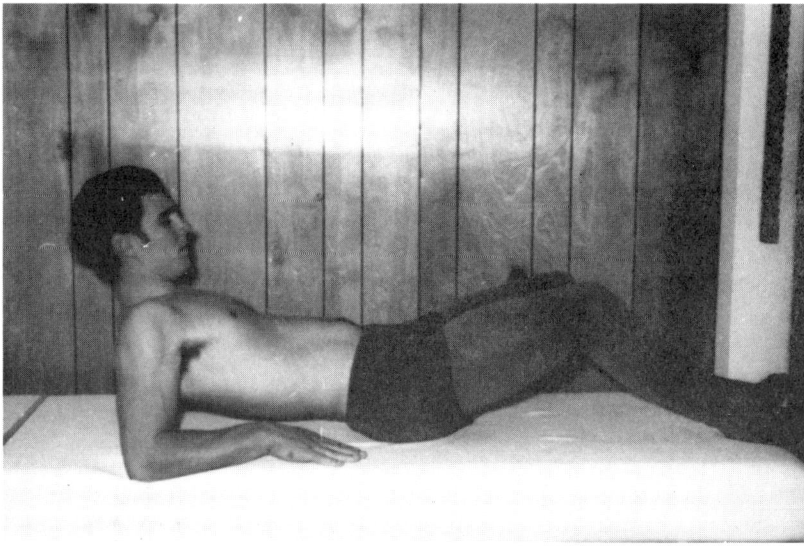

(Abdominals Relaxed)

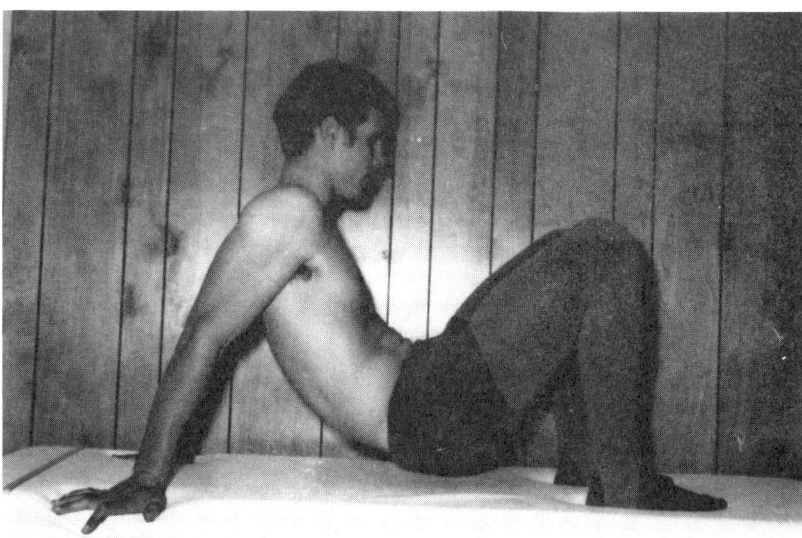

(Abdominals Contracted)

FIGURE 9 Moving from Head to Foot of Bed

keep the abdominals firm all the time until you are sitting up. First raise your head, shoulders, and arms until your abdominals are very firm. Then roll over on your side, bringing your feet off the side of the bed, and finally push your body up to a sitting position with your elbow and hand. As the feet go down along the side of the bed, the head and shoulders go up. The abdominals, being firm at all times, will not allow any rotation or lateral trunk flexion which would cause severe pain.

Returning from a sitting to a lying position, again the abdominals must be firm, with ribs down. As the head and shoulders go down to a side-lying position, the feet come up to the bed. Then you roll onto your back, your body moving as a whole unit.

SITTING-TO-STANDING—STANDING-TO-SITTING

Normally, when an individual gets up from a chair, bed, or any object that he may be sitting on, he bends at the waist, raises his head first, then his rib cage, and finally pushes with his feet. A patient with a low back strain experiences pain as soon as he begins to raise his rib cage, as at that time he begins to extend his back and initiate movement in the injured joint and tissue.

In order to get up without pain (figure 11), you must first drop your rib cage, round your back, and tighten the abdominal muscles firmly. Then place one foot in front of the other to increase balance. With your hands, push your weight forward over your feet and bend the knees forward, as if to kneel. When all the weight is over the legs, maintain your firm abdominal muscles and push up with your legs until you are standing. The harder you push with your legs, the more you slouch and tighten the abdominals. In this manner no motion takes place in the lumbar spine or low back and the movement is pain free.

When an individual normally moves from a standing to a sitting position (figure 12), he bends at the knees and hips. When he gets to the seat level he reaches for the seat with his buttocks. At this point he tilts the pelvis forward and arches his back, causing severe pain.

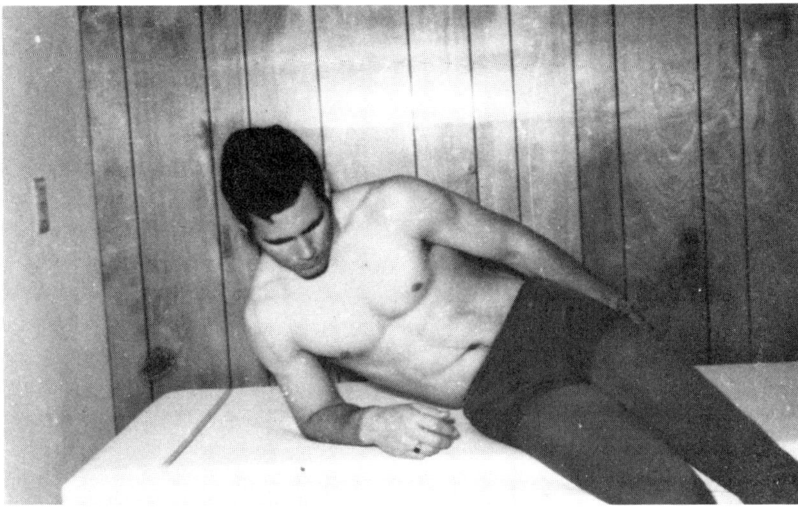

(Abdominals Relaxed)

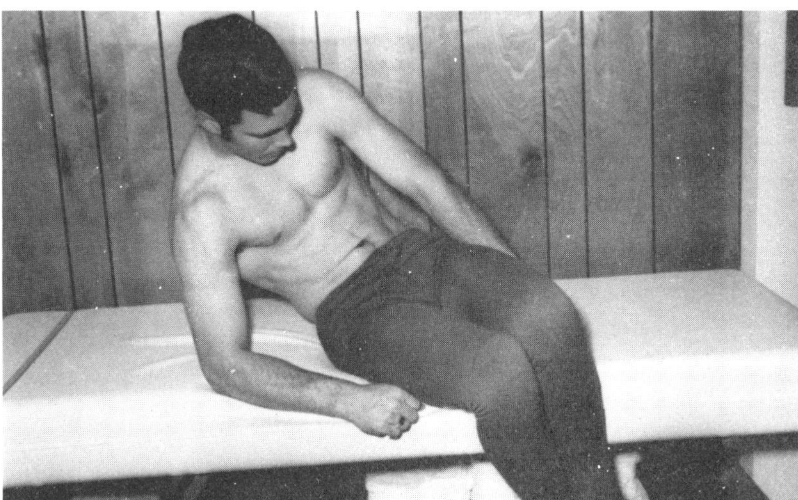

(Abdominals Contracted)

FIGURE 10 Moving from Lying to Sitting Position

FIGURE 11 Sitting-to-Standing

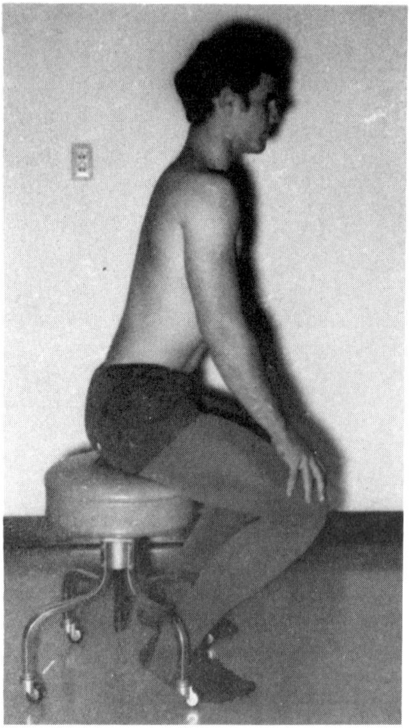

(Abdominals Relaxed)

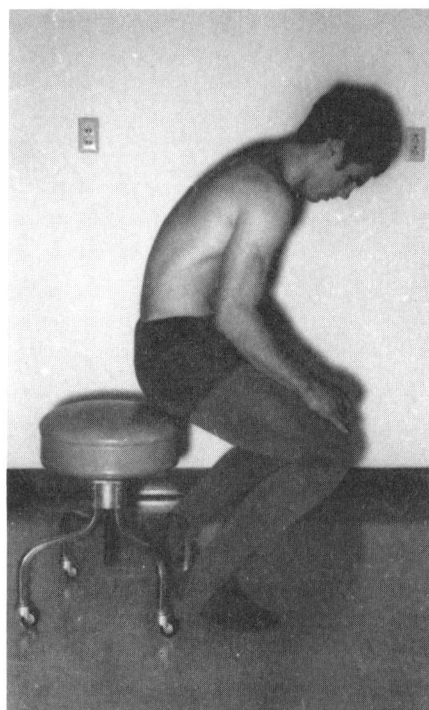

(Abdominals Contracted)

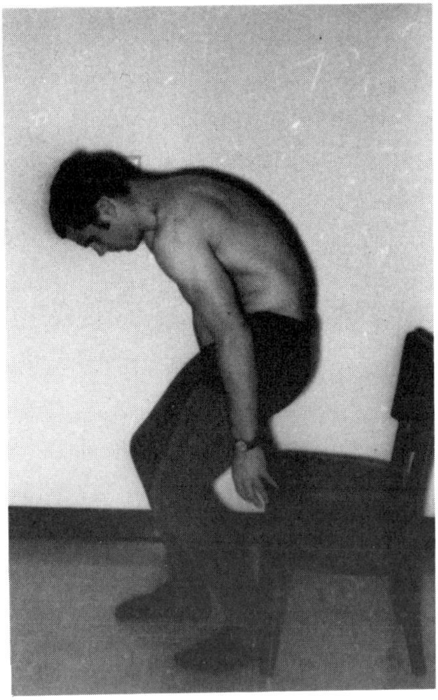

(Abdominals Contracted)

Figure 12 Standing-to-Sitting

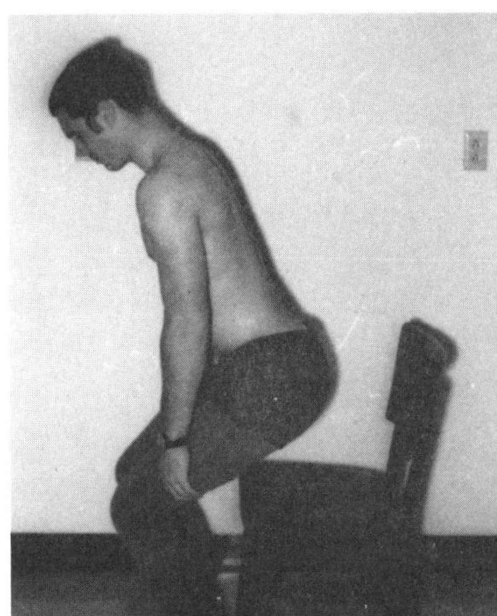

(Abdominals Relaxed)

To accomplish this movement without pain, you must drop your rib cage, round your back, and tighten your abdominals, keeping them firm at all times. The next move is to bend the knees forward, as if to kneel or sit on your heels. When the hips reach the seat level reach back for the seat with your hands and finally take your entire body into the seat as a unit. Again there is no movement or pain in the low back. You should note that the entire back is round when the abdominals are completely contracted, not straight. The buttocks will be underneath your body.

Sitting-to-standing and standing-to-sitting are two of the most important movements to master properly since so many activities of daily living are involved with these techniques. Some of these activities include getting up and down from a couch, chair, toilet, automobile, bed, and whatever other object a person may want to sit on or in. It is also the first movement of many other activities such as lifting, reaching, pushing, and pulling, as I will explain later.

STANDING

Once you push yourself up into a standing position it is most important that you maintain your low back in a strain-free position if you wish to prevent irritation and continue the healing process.

The most favorable position in standing is to keep the low back flat (figure 5). This can only be done with the abdominal muscles firm, pulling the rib cage down toward your abdomen and pulling your pubis up to your abdomen, and keeping your pelvis level. You should experience a feeling of sitting on a fence or wire with your upper back slouched.

If the hip flexors or muscles of the groin are too short you will tend to bend your knees in order to place yourself in this pain-free position. Many people have such tight hip flexors that it is impossible for them to stand in a strain-free position since they would have to bend their knees to an uncomfortable and strange-looking position. Tight hip flexors must be stretched out in order to stand in a strain-free position. These exercises will be discussed in the section on therapeutic exercise.

If you have to stand for any length of time as when ironing or working at a bench, placing one leg on a chair or stool will keep your back flat without maintaining your abdominal muscles firm.

When your low back is in the proper position you must then pull your shoulder blades back and down without lifting your chest or rib cage. If you lift your rib cage you will relax your abdominals, arch your back, and cause pain. (If you keep your ribs down, this will allow you to pull your chin in and place your head over your rib cage.) All these movements will give you an upright position of your entire trunk and head. Your entire spine should be straight.

If you are unable to place yourself in this position, you probably need further exercises for the shoulders and neck to increase flexibility. These also will be discussed later under therapeutic exercise.

WALKING

When a person walks he normally shifts his weight from one leg to the other. As he transfers his weight and then places all his weight on one leg momentarily, there is a considerable amount of movement in the low back. The movement consists of lateral flexion and rotation in the lumbar spine. Because of this movement pain is elicited in the low back by irritation of the injured joint. Since there is practically no rotation in the lumbar spine, a little movement can cause a lot of pain.

The abdominal muscles alone can prevent movement in the low back area when a person walks. When the abdominal muscles are contracted firmly, the rib cage, the lumbar spine, the dorsal spine, and the pelvis become fixed. The lumbar spine is fixed in a flattened position, placing the center of gravity of the upper trunk through the center of or anterior to the injured joint (figure 13).

FIGURE 13 Walking

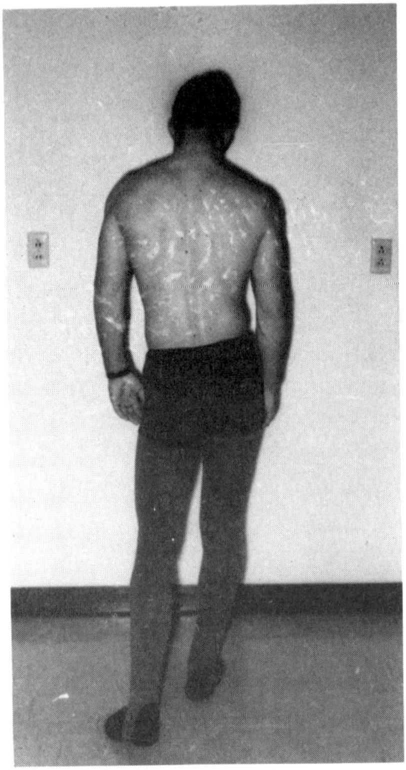

(Abdominals Relaxed)

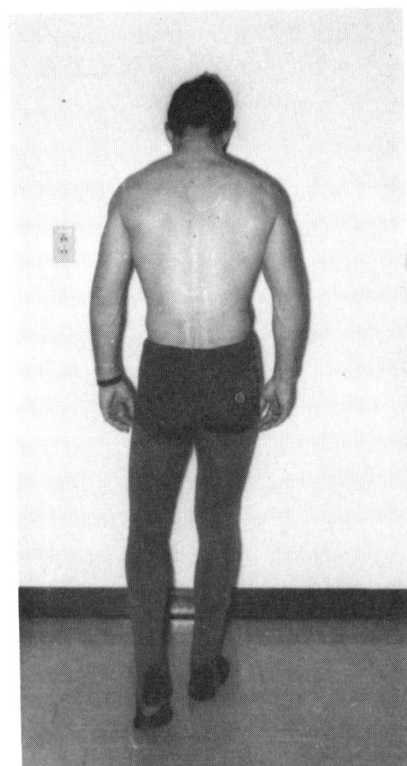

(Abdominals Contracted)

The abdominals act as a perfect brace since motion is completely eliminated. All movements of walking consequently take place in the lower extremities and pain is eliminated.

The amount of force needed by the abdominals is proportional to the amount of force needed to maintain stability. For example, it would take less force to walk with your hands free than it would if you had a suitcase in one hand.

STANDING-TO-SQUATTING

This movement is similar to standing-to-sitting, which was discussed earlier. The abdominals are contracted firmly. The knees are then allowed to bend forward as in kneeling. Incidentally, to maintain greater balance one foot should be placed ahead of the other, increasing the anterior posterior base. Continue to allow your knees to bend forward until you are sitting on the heel of your rear foot (figure 14).

You must not allow your abdominals to relax as most people do. If you do, the bottom of your pelvis will go backwards, creating an arch in your low back, and you will experience pain. You must keep your rib cage down and your back rounded with the abdominals.

SQUATTING-TO-STANDING

Returning from a squatting to a standing position is usually most painful for a person with a strained low back, simply because he has to lift his body weight against gravity.

The manner in which most people perform this movement begins with the raising of the head, then the shoulders, and then the rib cage. At this point, severe pain is experienced when the back muscles begin to arch the back. Finally, most people finish up by pushing with their legs.

If the abdominal muscles are contracted firmly, you may be able to raise your head, but it is impossible to lift the rib cage. Therefore, it is impossible to arch your back and create pain. Keeping your abdominal muscles firm, you simply push up with

Figure 14 Standing-to-Squatting

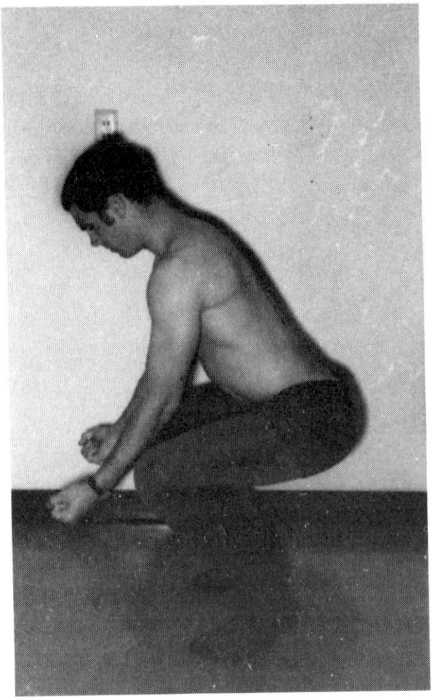

(Abdominals Relaxed)

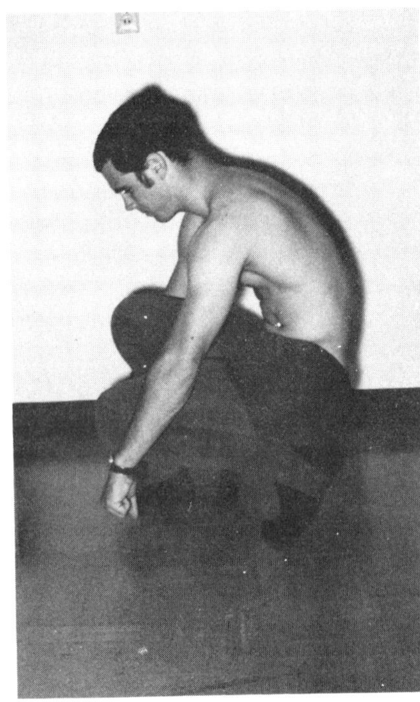

(Abdominals Contracted)

your legs. You will not experience any pain because there is no movement in the injured low back joint (figure 15).

BENDING AND RAISING AT THE HIPS

Many patients are unable to squat for many reasons. Some are much too heavy and their legs are too weak. Some have chronic knee injuries. Many people have occupations in which they must reach over tables to lift and are unable to bend their knees forward to squat.

It is possible to bend at the hips and lift without using your back. The most important factor again is to contract the abdominals, round your upper back, then bend over at the hip joints, keeping the legs straight (figure 16). There is no danger of hurting your back going down unless you either stop on the way down, relax your abdominals, and arch your back, or straighten your back with your back muscles. Once you do this, movement occurs in the low back, causing strain and pain.

Returning to a standing position after you have bent over becomes more difficult to accomplish without pain. The natural move is to raise the head and shoulders, but immediately you will experience pain. This you must never do. First, you must tighten the abdominal muscles so that you cannot lift your ribs. The next move is to squeeze your buttocks muscles firmly and pull yourself up with your hip muscles, with the only movement occurring in the hip joints. If movement is confined to the hip joints, you will not experience pain.

STANDING-TO-KNEELING—KNEELING-TO-STANDING

Many occupations, and housework especially, require work done in the low positions and there is a need for stability for a period of time. The kneeling position is ideal for this type of work. I believe it is essential that the kneeling take place on one knee only. While you are in the standing position, before kneeling, one foot should be placed at least two feet ahead of the other,

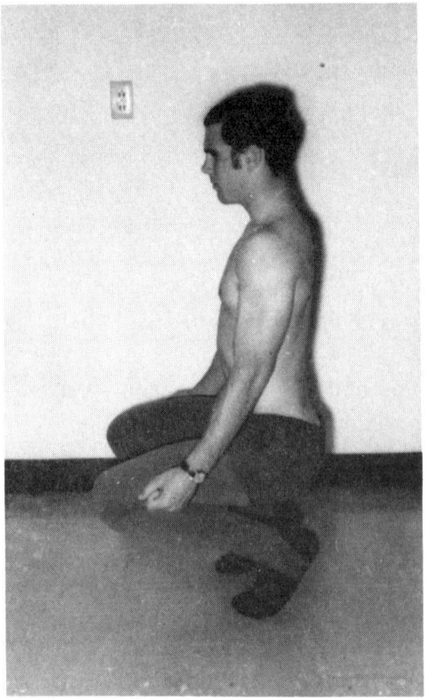

(Abdominals Relaxed)

FIGURE 15
Squatting-to-Standing

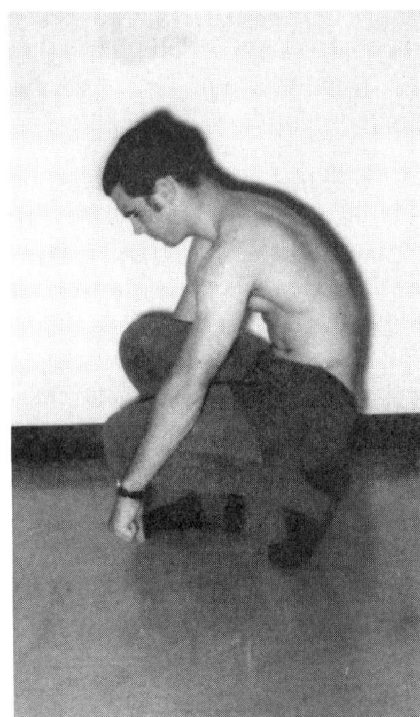

(Abdominals Contracted)

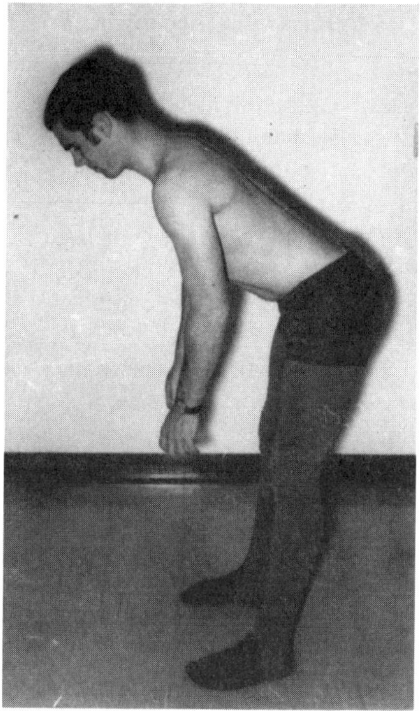

(Abdominals Relaxed)

FIGURE 16
Bending and Raising at the Hips

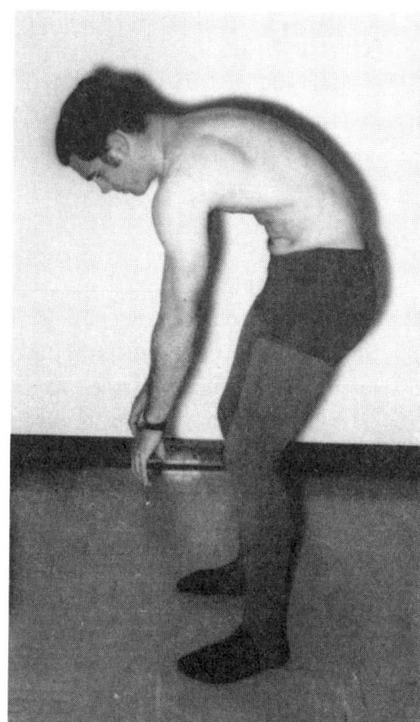

(Abdominals Contracted)

with your feet wide enough apart to establish a good base. Again, the most important thing is to contract your abdominal muscles firmly and then go forward and down on your rear knee. The thigh of the front leg should be against your chest and protecting your back, keeping it flat when you relax (figure 17). This is an excellent position for polishing, waxing, vacuuming floors, making beds, getting clothes out of dryers, and getting into a chest of drawers. Carpenters, plumbers, electricians, and painters can also get to low places without straining.

If your work requires force in this position, it is necessary that you contract your abdominals firmly so that you are free to use your shoulders, arms, and legs forcefully.

When returning to the standing position from a kneeling position, again keep your abdominals tight and push up and back with your legs.

If you are forced to kneel on both knees, you must maintain your abdominals firm and sit back on your heels. Don't relax your abdominals or you will raise your ribs and experience pain.

REACHING

Reaching overhead is one of the most difficult movements for anyone who has back pain. This is so because as one reaches overhead the rib cage automatically raises following the shoulders and arms. The raising of the rib cage arches the low back and causes pain, or places the low back in a vulnerable position. When force is applied by the arms in this position, the strain in the low back is multiplied and consequently there is pain.

Before reaching, the rib cage should be dropped completely as in slouching. Then the abdominal muscles should be contracted, maintaining the ribs in this position and locking the low back. Now, as you reach with your arms, while your abdominal muscles are firm, the ribs are unable to raise (figure 18). In this manner, the low back is maintained in a flat, locked position, and if it can't move, it can't be injured. The only areas of strain and movement will be in the shoulders and hip joints.

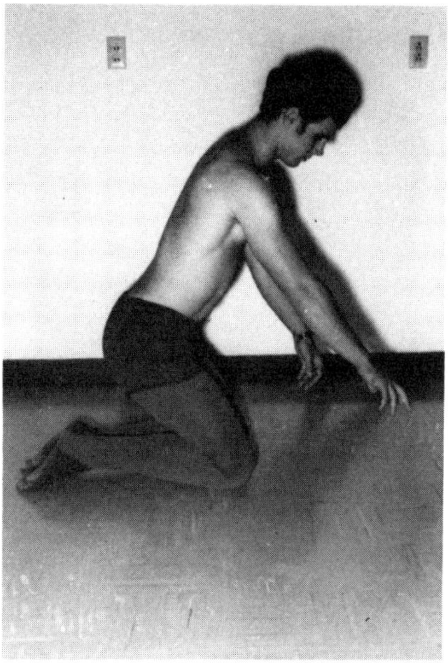

(Abdominals Relaxed)

FIGURE 17
Standing-to-Kneeling

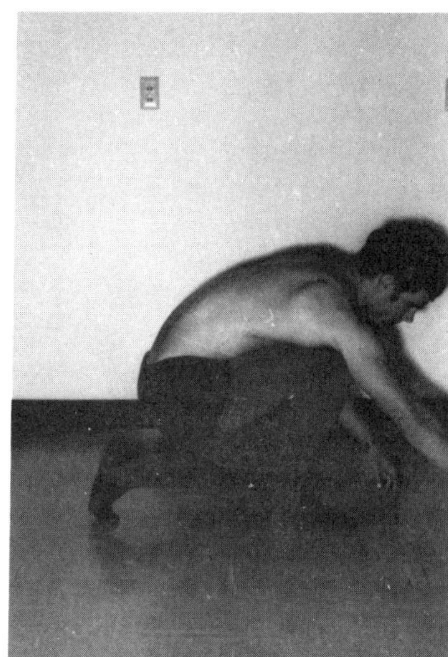

(Abdominals Contracted)

FIGURE 18 Reaching

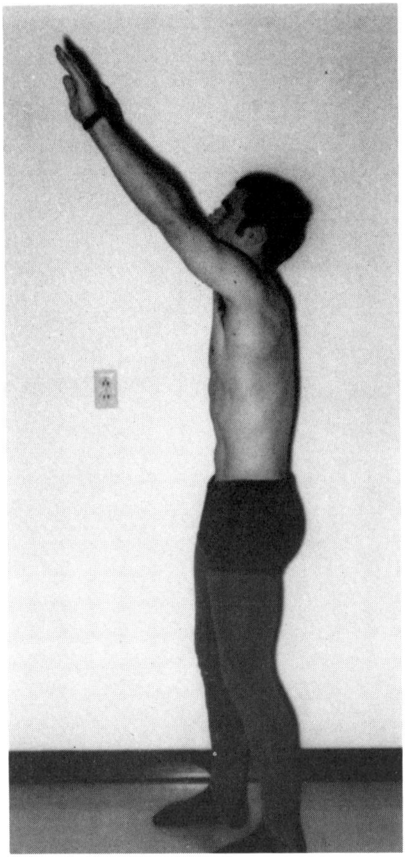

(Abdominals Contracted)

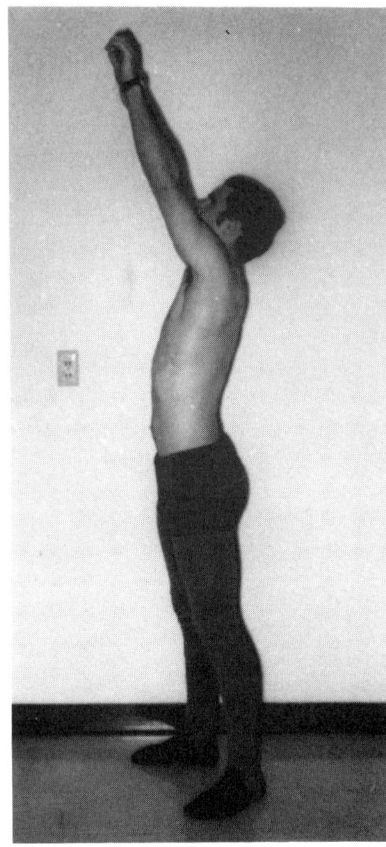

(Abdominals Relaxed)

If you cannot reach your objective properly, a stool or a ladder should be used so that you can reach properly.

When force is applied by the arms in a reaching position, the force of the abdominals must be increased proportionately to prevent movement in the low back. Only in this manner can you prevent strain and pain.

CLIMBING—ASCENDING

The average person does more climbing than he is aware of. A person with a back strain becomes very conscious of climbing stairs, hills, ladders, poles, or trees. His awareness is usually due to pain or fear of aggravating the pain or weakness that he has.

The reason for the increased pain when climbing is that the normal mechanics of climbing includes arching or extending the low back. Let us first analyze the normal manner of climbing.

Raising one leg up a normal step as in climbing stairs may cause slight discomfort, as there may be some side bending when the weight is all on one leg. The difficulty increases as we lift our entire body up the step. As we begin the climb, we raise our head and chest as we push down on the step with our lifting-forward leg and rise up on the toe of the back leg. When we raise the chest with our back muscles, we begin to arch the back, relax the abdominal muscles, and create a strain in the low back. We use our back muscles and raise our chest to lessen the strain on our leg muscles by changing the resistance on the lever of our hip and ankle joints, thereby allowing us to climb with much less effort. We also tend to raise the chest as we come up on the toe of the back leg, in order to keep our balance and distribute the strain over both legs. Since the low back lever is injured in the person with a back strain, he must keep from using the low back extensor muscles. The only way that this can be done is by contracting the abdominal muscles firmly and locking the low back joint.

When climbing, the abdominal muscles must be contracted firmly before the transferring of weight from the back leg to the front leg. By maintaining the contraction, the back is unable to arch and all the effort is placed on the muscles of the hip, knee, ankle joints and abdomen (figure 19).

If you keep your abdominal muscles contracted forcefully, you will note much greater strain on your forward leg. This is the result of keeping the center of gravity of your body more forward when the knee is flexed at ninety degrees. There also will be less strain on the back leg.

When your abdominals are relaxed, the center of gravity is divided between both legs, distributing the strain more equally on each leg. However, the low back is in a strained position and the strain is increased as the body is lifted up. Consequently, keep your abdominals forcefully contracted and your weight forward.

DESCENDING

Descending stairs, hills, and other elevations may be more difficult and painful than climbing. This is so because, in a way, we fall down a step and catch ourselves with one of our legs. During this process we tend to keep our center of gravity behind our forward leg to keep from falling down the stairs or on our face. We keep our weight back by arching our back. With the back arched in a strained position, we drop down a step in a jarring manner, which may be very painful and is certainly aggravating even if we drop down slowly.

To descend without straining the low back, you first must prevent arching the back by contracting the abdominal muscles to keep from jarring the spine. In descending you must lower your body down with the back leg. You continue lowering your body down until the front foot is on the lower step; then you transfer your weight from the back leg to the front leg (figure 20).

The movement of lowering your weight gives you a feeling as though you are about to sit on your back leg and the step that you are descending from.

By using this technique you have complete control of your body at all times. All the effort is in the legs and there is no need or tendency to arch the back or jar it.

FIGURE 19 Ascending (Climbing)

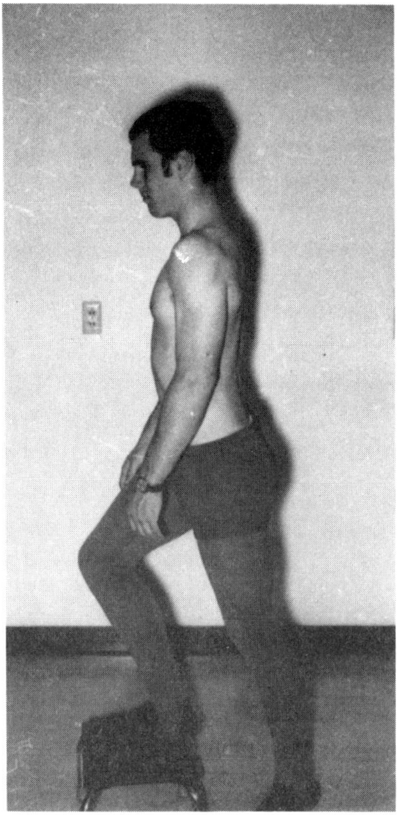

(Abdominals Relaxed)

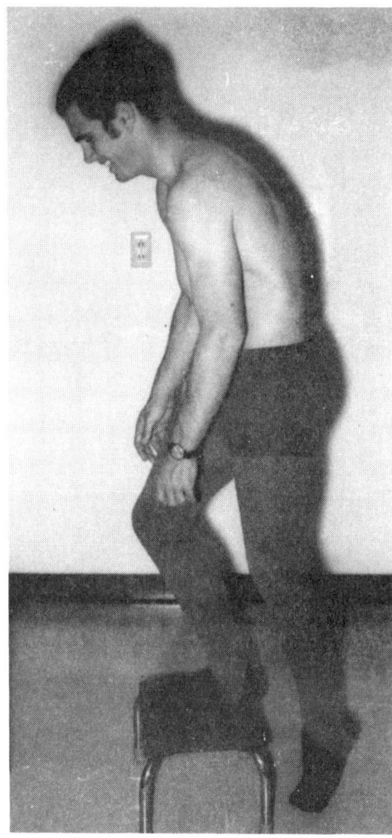

(Abdominals Contracted)

FIGURE 20 Descending

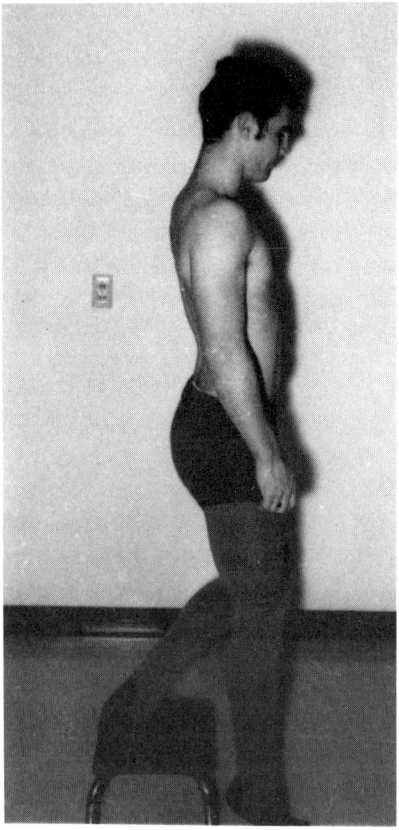

(Abdominals Relaxed)

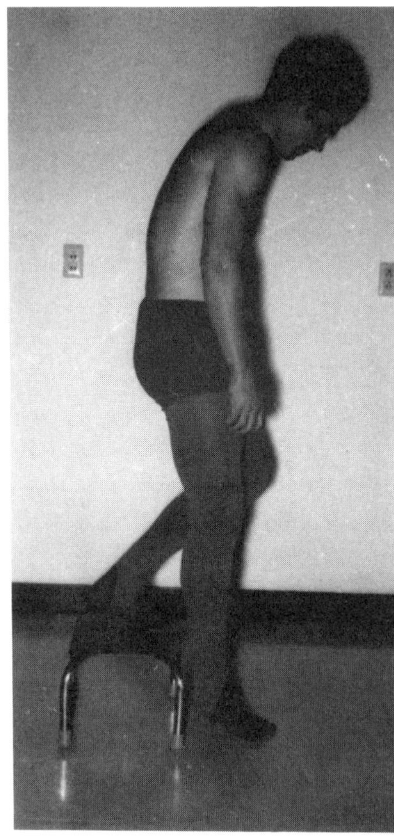

(Abdominals Contracted)

RUNNING

Running may be most aggravating or impossible for a person with a strained back because of the tremendous jarring and kicking involved.

The natural tendency in running is to arch the back considerably to keep from falling on your face from the forward momentum developed with speed. With the back in a strained position, each time the ground is hit and a forceful kick forward is made, the strain is multiplied and the pain is proportionately multiplied.

The only way running can be done without pain is to straighten the low back joint and keep it straight with your abdominal muscles (figure 21). You will have the same protection as an athlete has who tapes a sprained ankle before running. The taping prevents movement in the direction of the strain and consequently prevents pain. The abdominals do the same in running.

Your style of running will have to change as you will have to round your back considerably and keep your hips tucked under when you contract your abdominals completely.

If pain is experienced with this technique, chances are the strain is too acute, with considerable tenderness and swelling in and around the injured tissue. Running should then be discouraged until it can be done without pain.

TWISTING

Twisting is another basic movement of the body. Most twisting in the spine takes place in the dorsal or mid spine. In the lumbar spine or low back, there is very little rotation. Therefore, a forceful twist or a forceful strain when the body is twisted can very easily injure the low back. Consequently, a patient with a low back injury or back pain can very easily aggravate his condition or feel intense pain with a slight twist as when one is turning in bed or getting into an automobile. Because of the lack of rotation in the low back, immediate stress is placed on the

Figure 21 Running

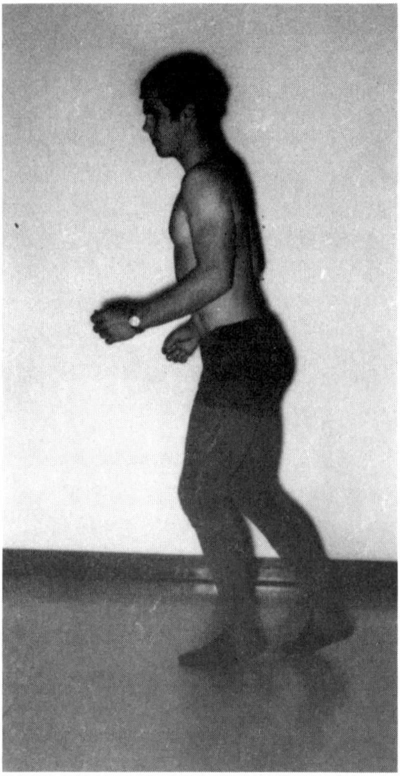

(Abdominals Relaxed)

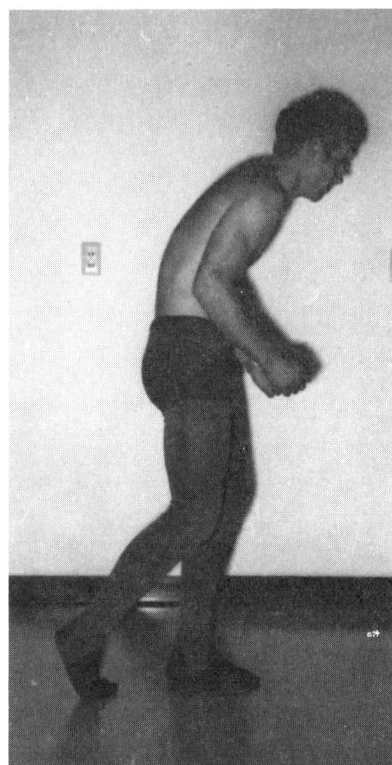

(Abdominals Contracted)

vertebrae and the supporting tissues, causing pain when twisting occurs.

To prevent rotation or twisting in the low back, you must again drop your rib cage and contract your abdominal muscles. Now, if you try to twist your body to the right or left in the standing position, you must twist in the hip joints. If the knees are slightly flexed, some rotation takes place at the knees (figure 22).

When the abdominals are firm, rotation in the dorsal or mid spine is prevented. Consequently, total rotation of your body becomes limited. However, there is enough rotation in the hip joints

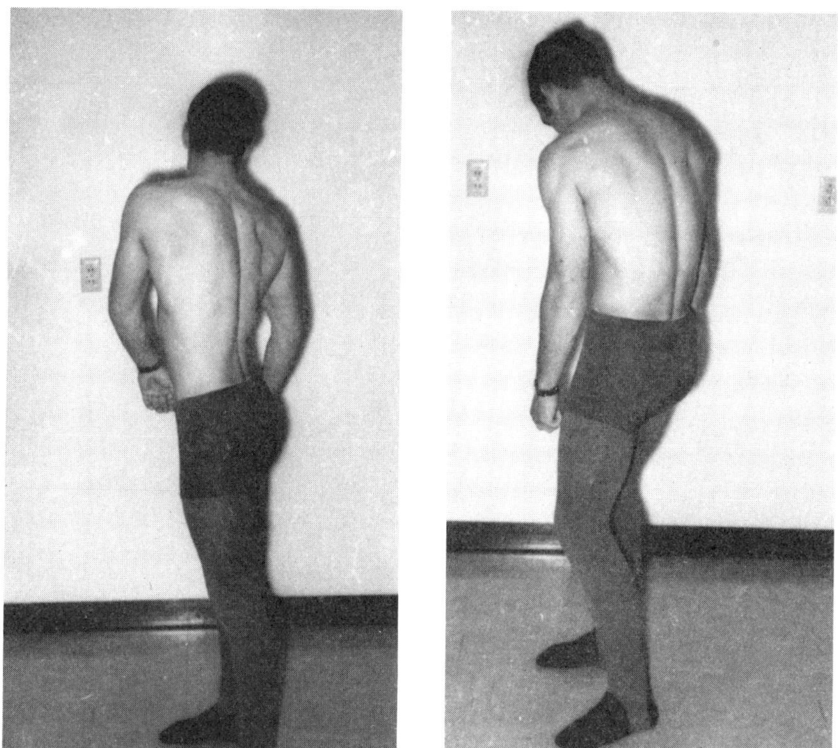

(Abdominals Relaxed) (Abdominals Contracted)

FIGURE 22 Twisting

to perform almost all activities to the right or left. If you are unable to rotate the hips sufficiently, you should pivot on your feet or turn your entire body, rather than twist improperly. Here again, if your abdominal muscles prevent twisting or movement in the low back, pain will not be experienced and the injured tissue will be protected for further healing.

Chapter IV

BASIC MOVEMENTS WITH INCREASED STRAIN

LIFTING

Most back injuries occur after forceful, and at times not so forceful, lifting. Consequently, learning to lift properly is most significant in allowing a back injury to heal as well as in preventing future injuries.

Lifting is similar to getting up from a chair to a standing position, or moving from a squatting to a standing position. However, much lifting is also done in the standing position, as in lifting objects overhead.

To lift objects from the floor to a standing position, you first get into a proper squatting position as was described earlier. Before you lift the object, you must contract your abdominal muscles firmly and lock your back. Now, as you lift, you must keep your back locked and push your body and the object up with your legs and your abdominal muscles (figure 23). If you relax your abdominals slightly or raise your rib cage while you are lifting, you will experience pain. The heavier the object, the greater will be the strain on the abdominal muscles.

When lifting in a standing position, the object must be held close to the body, since most of the lifting will be done by shoulders and arm muscles. The object should be pushed up overhead only as high as the arms can reach without raising the rib

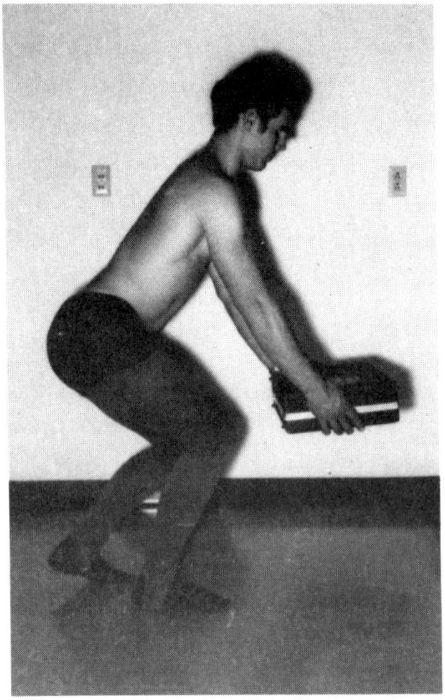

(Abdominals Relaxed)

FIGURE 23 Lifting

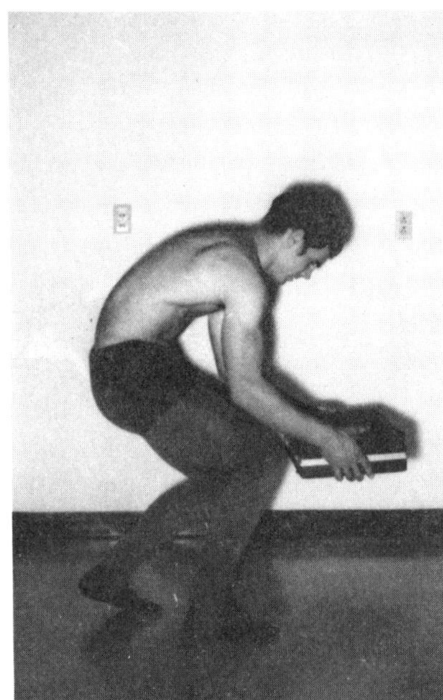

(Abdominals Contracted)

cage or releasing the abdominal muscles. The low back must be straight, supported, and immovable throughout the entire act of lifting the object.

If you find yourself bending at the waist with your legs straight, don't ever come back up the same way that you went down to lift the object. When rising from such a position, first bend your knees forward until your pelvis is perpendicular to the ground with your buttocks under you and your back rounded. With your abdominals firm, push yourself up with your legs and don't raise your ribs until your legs are straight again. In this manner you will prevent motion in your low back and thereby prevent an injury or aggravation.

PUSHING OBJECTS

Everyone must push objects during the day. A housewife will push furniture such as beds, couches, and many other objects around a home. A man will push lawnmowers, automobiles, heavy doors, and many other objects many times a day, depending on his occupation.

Once again the same principle applies that I have been emphasizing throughout this book. If you can keep the injured joint from moving, you will not aggravate the injury and you will not create any additional injury to this area.

First, you must balance yourself by placing one foot a step or so ahead of the other, depending on how forceful a push is needed. The farther apart the feet are, the more stability is developed. Secondly, you contract or tighten your abdominal muscles, flattening your low back, and bring the ribs down toward your pubis and abdomen (figure 24). Keeping your back in this position, you can push as hard as you want without injuring your back. You can bend your knees as much as you like, but you must never relax your abdominal muscles and allow your low back to arch, for if you do this you must use the injured joint. If the force is greater than the injured joint can tolerate, further aggravation or more serious injury may result.

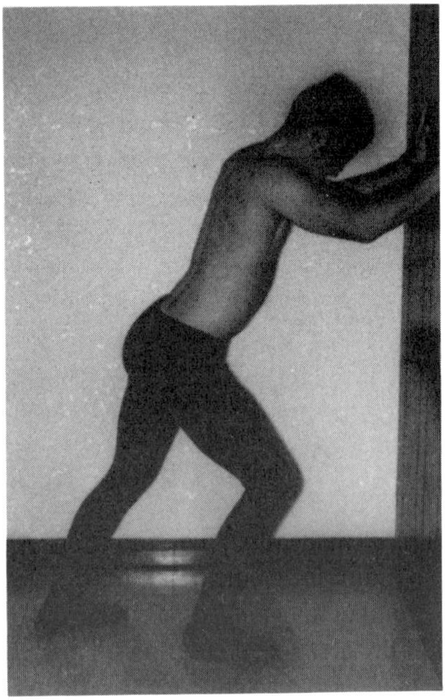

(Abdominals Relaxed)

FIGURE 24 Pushing

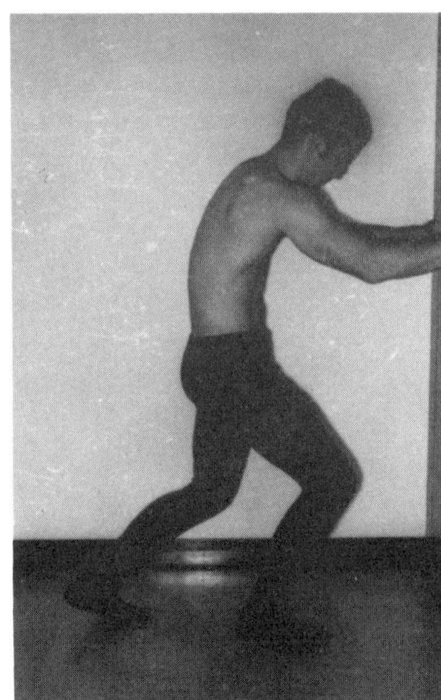

(Abdominals Contracted)

One further note: as you push harder, you might tighten your abdominals harder. The abdominal force must be proportionate to the force of the push.

PULLING

Pulling is similar to pushing, except more dangerous, as there is a strong tendency to extend or arch the back if it is done improperly.

In pulling, you lean away from the object. To lessen the danger, keep one foot considerably farther ahead of the other. The difficulty in pulling properly is that it is very unnatural to keep your abdominal muscles firm and at the same time pull back with your buttocks muscles, using the hip joints as the fulcrum. The tendency is to use the back muscles with the hip muscles, using both the low back and the hip joints as fulcrums, thereby expending less effort.

Assume the same position as in pushing. Maintain the firm abdominals and use the opposite muscle groups that you used in pushing (figure 25). Pulling by using your legs as in walking backwards may help to keep the abdominals tight and avoid using the back muscles.

DRESSING ACTIVITIES

To many patients with back pain, dressing becomes a great problem, as normally there is a considerable amount of motion in the low back when one is dressing.

Acute cases should put on pants, or panties, socks or stockings, and shoes in a back-lying position in bed. They can then bend in the hip joints. They will probably be able to do most, if not all, of the dressing alone. With the back supported by the bed, there is not too much chance of injury. When they stand up they can pull up their pants the remainder of the way. Shirts and other upper body clothing can be put on safely in a sitting position.

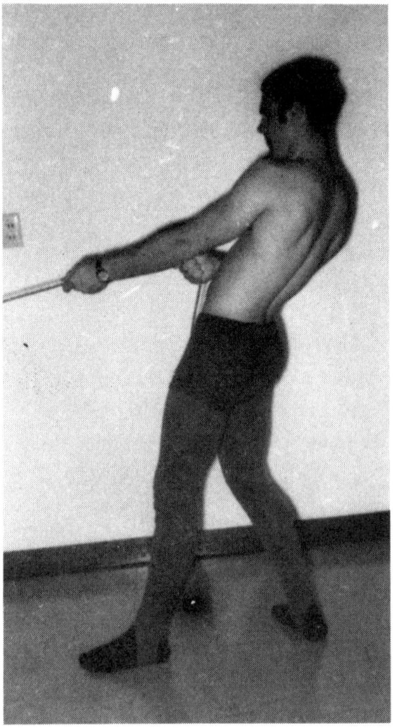

(Abdominals Relaxed)

FIGURE 25 Pulling

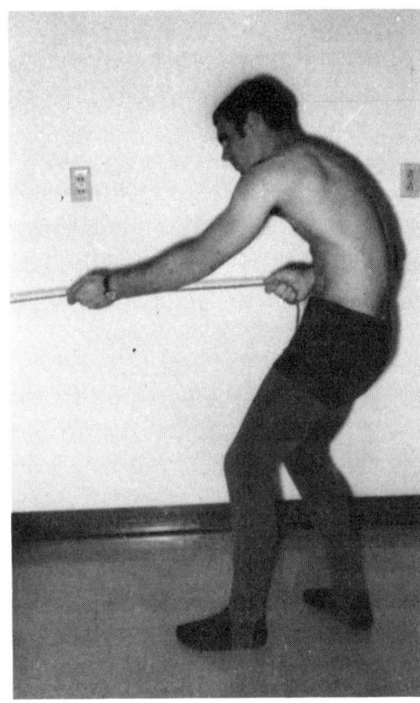

(Abdominals Contracted)

One should never attempt to put his or her pants, socks, or shoes on in a standing position, as he will have to balance on one leg in order to perform the activity. This takes good balance and flexibility which he may not have with one weak leg. Therefore, he may lose his balance and create motion in the injured joint and again aggravate or produce further injury.

Tightening the abdominal muscles can be applied in dressing activities as in the other activities which we have discussed. All other joints can be used freely if you can maintain the low back in a stable, flat position by the use of the abdominal muscles.

SEXUAL INTERCOURSE

One of the most important functions of human beings is sexual intercourse, which is necessary for a happy married life. Being unable to perform this function not only affects the individual with the back strain but also his mate, who may be in psychological pain.

Because of the closeness of the bodies during intercourse pain would be caused by arching the low back. This would occur only when the top of the pelvis is tipped forward, or during the extreme withdrawal phase of performing. During the inserting phase the abdominals and hip extensor muscles are brought into action forcefully tipping the pelvis backward and flattening the back. The inserting phase should not cause pain and could be a beneficial exercise for low back strain as it has a tendency to flatten the back and strengthen the abdominal muscles.

The best position for intercourse is in the back-lying position with both knees flexed and feet flat. The low back is completely flattened and the back is in a strain-free position.

If the abdominals are contracted firmly and maintained during the withdrawal phase, it is impossible to arch the back and cause pain or strain. It is only when you relax your abdominals and withdraw by using your back extensor muscles and arch your back that you will have pain. By keeping the abdominals firm on the withdrawal phase all movement occurs in the hip joints. Generally, you may keep your abdominals firm, maintaining the low back in the best position, and thus prevent movement in the low back in both phases of intercourse.

After learning the technique and control, other positions may be mastered. Any position in which the abdominals can be completely contracted and the hip joints are free to move should be successful and pain free.

PREGNANCY

Most women in the last few months of pregnancy have considerable difficulty with the low back. As the baby grows the weight in front of the low back increases, changing the center of gravity. To compensate for this increased weight anteriorly, the mother must tilt her rib cage and shoulders backwards with her back muscles to keep her weight or center of gravity over her feet. Otherwise she would fall forward.

The low back curve increases as the shoulders and ribs go backward. If the abdominals are relaxed, the weight of the baby is also pulling the apex of the lumbar curve forward. With the abdominals relaxed the back extensors are the only muscles that keep the mother upright. With an increased low back curve and the back muscles holding all the anterior weight up, there is a great strain placed on the last joint of the low back as the back muscles pull on this fulcrum.

To eliminate a backache due to pregnancy or to keep it to a minimum much can be done. The low back curve can be lessened; the abdominal muscles can be strengthened. Flexibility of the hip, shoulder, and ankle joints can be restored. Finally, and most important of all, the mother can be taught how to use her abdominal muscles to prevent stress and strain in the low back.

Once flexibility and strength are restored, the mother must contract the abdominal muscles in the standing position, keeping the child on top of her pelvis and not allowing the baby to hang in front tipping the pelvis forward. By contracting the abdominal muscles the pelvis is tipped backwards flattening the low back and the baby is being pushed in on top of the pelvis.

The exercises explained in this book can apply to pregnant women who need to restore flexibility and strengthen the abdominals. The techniques of functional training using the abdominals discussed in this book also apply to pregnant women if they would like to prevent stress and strain in the low back and have much less difficulty during pregnancy and the period following.

WORKING

Up to this point we have discussed all the basic movements of the body that are necessary in performing the activities of daily living such as getting up and down, reaching, and so forth. You should master these basic movements.

Regardless of what kind of work a person has to do, he is usually performing some task with his hands and legs as in plumbing, carpentry, electronics, manual labor, and many, many other types of work. If people do not use their bodies physically in performing some type of work, they would then use their brains or both their minds and their bodies. Most jobs involve both, with emphasis greater on either the brain or body depending on the work and the situation.

From what I can analyze, the back itself is unproductive; it is unable to accomplish anything. The legs propel you to the job and the arms or legs, or both, perform the task at hand. However, the arms and legs are attached to the back and consequently everything we do affects the back. This applies to all types of work as well as all activities of daily living.

The important fact to keep in mind is not so much what your hands and legs may be doing but what is happening to your low back while you are using your arms and legs.

If the low back can be maintained in a straight-backed and immovable position you will not experience any pain or discomfort while performing any type of work. This can only be done by completely contracting the abdominal muscles and maintaining stability while using your arms and legs for whatever work you wish. Only in this way can you prevent extension or movement in the weak and injured joint.

If you do not contract your abdominal muscles, it is most likely that the joint will be in an unfavorable position and in a partial strain. When one uses his arms and legs this strain is multiplied since the arms and legs are attached to the spine and must affect the low back, resulting in movement of the injured joint and constant irritation.

There are some jobs or professions that cannot be performed with a weak back. Any job which requires extension of the spine such as tumbling, professional football, or circus stunts could not possibly be performed without pain until the injury is healed and the back is naturally strengthened. However, these types of work are not too common.

Jobs which include reacting to other people or machines may be more difficult to master. However, when most activities of daily living, or the basic movements discussed earlier, are mastered, proper reactions will become automatic after a while.

RECREATION AND SPORTS

Most recreational activities are performed by your arms and legs. The legs propel and the arms perform. However, the danger of recreational activities is that most activities are social and include other people. In this type of situation one must react to another person's action. Depending on the type of activity, reaction must be done quickly and instinctively in many situations. When the movement involves extension of the spine or a sudden twist to a weakened, tender joint, pain is experienced, irritation and aggravation result.

As I have explained throughout this book, any activity can be performed without pain or aggravation if movement in the injured joint can be prevented. Here again, the only way that you can prevent extension and twisting of the low back is by contracting your abdominal muscles completely before performing the activity. Consequently your arms and legs are free to react or perform.

I would recommend that individual types of recreational

activities be mastered first, since the activity can be completely controlled by the performer. Some of these activities are golfing, bowling, swimming, fishing, hunting, gardening, and many others. These activities can be performed without movement in the low back. Then you can slowly begin to train yourself in team activities such as volleyball, softball, handball, basketball, tennis, and others.

In all recreational activities all the basic movements discussed earlier are involved. Some activities include more twisting or reaching, while others include more squatting and standing. The only difference between activities of daily living and recreational activities is that the former are necessary and the latter are for fun.

Some activities are more difficult to do properly than others because of the greater tendency to arch the back. For example, while swimming the crawl stroke, the tendency is to hold the head up out of the water. By raising the head you tend to arch your back, which results in movement in the low back and subsequent irritation. Playing volleyball includes a great amount of reaching over the head. This movement tends to arch the back. You should only participate in activities that you can perform properly by fixing your low back with your abdominal muscles. As your habits improve, you can become more involved in more difficult activities.

Chapter V

USE OF ABDOMINALS IN OTHER CONDITIONS

OTHER DISEASES AND INJURIES TO THE LOW BACK

There are other problems of the low back besides strains and sprains. Osteoarthritis, multiple sclerosis, cancer of the spine, and many other conditions are possible but are not nearly as common as the low back strain.

Many of these conditions create weakness of the supporting structures in the low back. There may also be present severe tenderness and swelling. With such conditions and complications, movement of the low back joints produces severe pain.

It has been my experience that teaching patients with these conditions to use their abdominal muscles properly before movement lessens the severity of the pain considerably. The abdominal muscles support the joints and prevent movement in the low back, as described throughout this book. A considerable degree of discomfort and suffering caused by movement can be prevented by this technique.

BACK SURGERY—LAMINECTOMY

I believe that many people have poor to fair results from surgery for two reasons. First, in spite of the repair by a laminectomy, muscles and ligaments that support the joint may be too weak. Either the cause of the weakness has not been eliminated or the tissue has not had a sufficient opportunity to heal and strengthen because of constant irritation. The entire problem has not been eliminated; the disc may be repaired, but the back strain is still present. If post-surgically you continue to use your back improperly and the back is weak, the pain goes on. Secondly, the back supporting tissue may be strong; however, the improper use of the back may be constantly irritating the repaired and inflamed tissue and preventing the tissue from healing.

By using the abdominal muscles properly, as described in this book, you will stop the straining, and the weakened tissue can heal and strengthen. By using the abdominal muscles properly you prevent irritating movement, allowing the tissue irritated by the surgery to heal.

BACK SURGERY—FUSION

Once your back is fused and you continue to use your back as you did before, i.e., constantly arching it in every activity, you are constantly attempting to break your fusion. You are also straining the joint above and below the fusion because of the loss of flexibility caused by the fusion.

The purpose of the fusion is to prevent movement in the joint and maintain it in a certain position. By contracting your abdominal muscles properly you flatten the low back, preventing movement, and you are now working with the fusion instead of against it.

The exercise of pulling both knees up on the chest should not be done once the low back has been fused. This exercise may break or weaken a fusion. Instead, pulling one knee up to the chest at a time without towels under the hips will increase hip joint flexion, which is necessary. The more flexibility you have in the hip joints, the less chance there is of straining the low back.

If surgery must be done such as in the case of a ruptured or herniated disc or a fusion, maximum flexibility of the spine and hips should be first reached. The patient should also be taught proper posture and functional training techniques as described in this book.

If the patient is properly trained in functional training, post-surgery is much less difficult. Many patients have great difficulty moving in bed and getting up the first time following surgery. This is because every move they make either strains the low back or irritates it. By using the abdominal muscles properly, as described, the patient should be able to move almost without discomfort except for the increased pressure caused by the contracting abdominals.

It is much wiser if a patient can move himself in bed and get up without assistance, as he is more sensitive to his condition and has better control over his movement than someone who is assisting and not in coordination with his movement.

Chapter VI

PREVENTION OF RECURRING BACK PAIN

Mastering the use of your body with your abdominal muscles will not only place and keep your low back joint in a position to heal completely, but if you continue to use your abdominals properly, it will be impossible to reinjure the joint in the same manner as it was injured previously. Most people with a back problem continue to have recurrences, for when they are in pain they favor the back until it heals to a pain-free degree. Then they return to their same old ways and irritating habits. They gradually weaken the structures to the point of pain once again. It becomes a vicious cycle.

By maintaining your flexibility and by the proper use of your abdominals you can prevent recurrence of back pain. As time goes by the supporting tissues should be getting stronger instead of weaker. You will also prevent a considerable amount of osteoarthritic changes.

HABITS

You will make many mistakes while learning to use your abdominal muscles properly. However, you will be making less than you did in the past, and you will continue to make less each day.

The important thing is to be honest with yourself. If you know you are standing in the wrong position, correct yourself immediately. Eventually you will find yourself making less mistakes and less corrections.

If you know you are doing something wrong and you don't correct yourself you will never change your habits, and I believe that you will continue to have difficulty with your back.

Once your habits become fixed it is difficult to lose them, since they will feel natural. Then when you do an activity improperly it will feel unnatural and you will become aware of it immediately. At this time you can say that you have mastered your back.

You must look at your back problem over a long-range plan. It takes time for ligaments and muscles to strengthen. The important thing is that your back is getting stronger each day, each week, each month, each year.

Remember also that you are not only interested in getting over your present problem but you are going to prevent recurrences of the present problem and prevent any chance of causing another injury to your back.

Chapter VII

THERAPEUTIC EXERCISES

I believe the main purpose of exercising is to increase flexibility by stretching shortened muscles and ligaments. The increased flexibility then allows you to place your bones in a position in which you can eliminate the stress and strain on the injured tissue. Other purposes of exercise would include strengthening weakened muscles and stretching adhesions which may have developed from the injury.

LUMBAR FLEXION (figure 26)

Let's consider the flexibility of the low back. In order to eliminate stress and strain from the lower back all the joints must be straight and the low back should appear flat. Most people find this difficult to do because of the lack of flexion in the low back, and especially in the last joint that moves. The reason this flexibility is lost is because all basic movements, when done naturally, arch the back or extend the joints. Over the years you gradually increase your extension range and lose the flexion range, resulting in a swayback.

The first exercise is to test for flexion flexibility in the low back. In a back-lying position with your knees flexed and feet flat on the surface you are lying on, place a couple of folded towels under your hips. Keep the towels below the low back pain area. You may also place a couple of pillows under your feet.

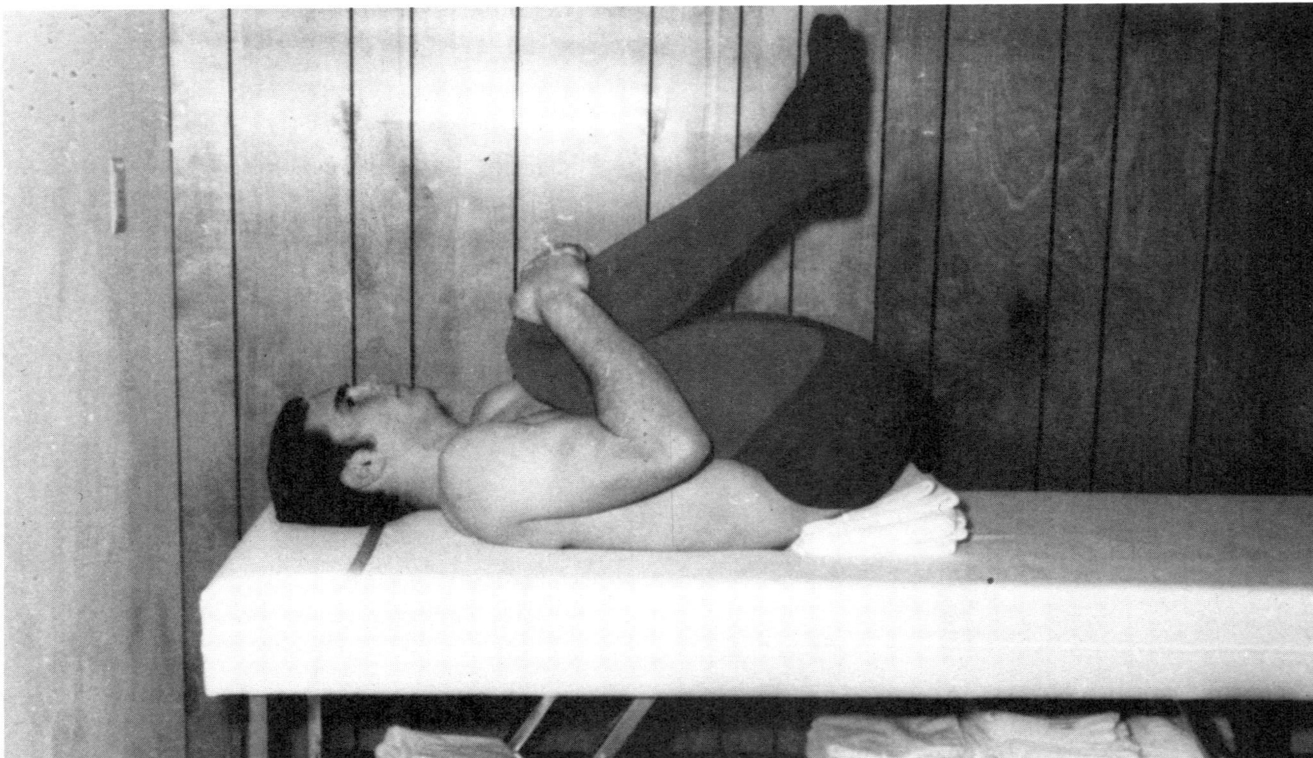

FIGURE 26 Lumbar Flexion

Now you are in the starting position and ready to begin the first exercise.

First, bring the leg with the least amount of pain up to your chest as far as is possible without aggravating the pain in your back or leg. The leg will stabilize your back and allow the affected leg to come up without pain. If pain is still experienced, raise your head and shoulders off the table first. This will stabilize your low back; then you can raise the unaffected side or leg without strain or pain. Once your unaffected leg is up as far as possible without pain, hold the knee firmly, keeping the low back flat, and then bring the other knee to your chest until you have both knees in your hands. Now relax your abdominal muscles, allowing your low back to drop down and your hips to raise. Pull both knees toward your chin or chest very slowly until you feel a stretch in the low back or the first sign of pain. This completes the stretching. In returning to the starting position, continue to hold on to the unaffected leg, allowing the affected leg to go down to the starting position, being constantly aware of keeping the low back flat with the unaffected leg on your chest. Once the affected leg is down, slowly let the unaffected leg down to the starting position. If pain is experienced at any time during the return, raise the head and shoulders off the table or surface and then proceed as described above. Raising the head and shoulders again will help to stabilize the low back with the contraction of the abdominal muscles.

If the low back muscles are tight and painful, this exercise will cause a stretching feeling or aggravate the pain if the pull is too forceful. Also the knees will not go up on the chest. If there is no tightness the knees will go up toward the chin and the thighs will be on the chest, stopping further movement and stretching. If this is so, this exercise will be of no value except that the completely flexed position may feel good because the joints in the low back are placed in a position of the least amount of strain. If the hip joints are extremely flexible, this exercise can aggravate the condition by overstretching the hip joints, and it should not be done.

STRETCHING HIP FLEXORS

Once you are able to get your knees on your chest without pain and without any stretch feeling in the low back, you are now ready for another low back exercise, which is stretching of the groins or hip flexors. These are the muscles that go from your low back through your groin and attach to the top of your thigh. When they contract they bring your thigh up toward your abdomen as when going upstairs. If these muscles are too short it is impossible to stand with your back flat and your legs straight. Most people with tightened or shortened hip flexors are sway-backed and the only way they can flatten the low back is when they bend their knees when they sit, or when they bend over considerably (as many old people and young people do with badly aching backs). This is the position in which you see most acute back patients walk into a doctor's office or the hospital. They do this to relieve the pain by flattening their low backs.

Stretching of the hip flexors is started from the same position as stretching the low back in the first exercise. Lie down with folded towels under your pelvis and pillows under your feet. The first movement is to pull the unaffected knee up on your chest and hug it tightly with both arms so that the low back is completely flexed and immovable. Now straighten out the other leg and let it hang slightly out to the side, as the muscles extend from the center of the back to the hip joint at a slight angle. You should feel a stretch in the groin of the lower leg (figure 27). Do not let go of the leg on your chest in order to straighten the lower leg. This will only allow your low back to come up and the injured joint may get strained.

Do not let go of the leg on your chest until you bring the lower leg up to a flexed position and your foot is flat on the surface.

If the lower leg (thigh) straightens out and is parallel to your low back, chances are that your hip flexors are not shortened and this exercise would not be necessary. In fact, it may strain your hip joint if you continue stretching after the thigh is parallel to your low back.

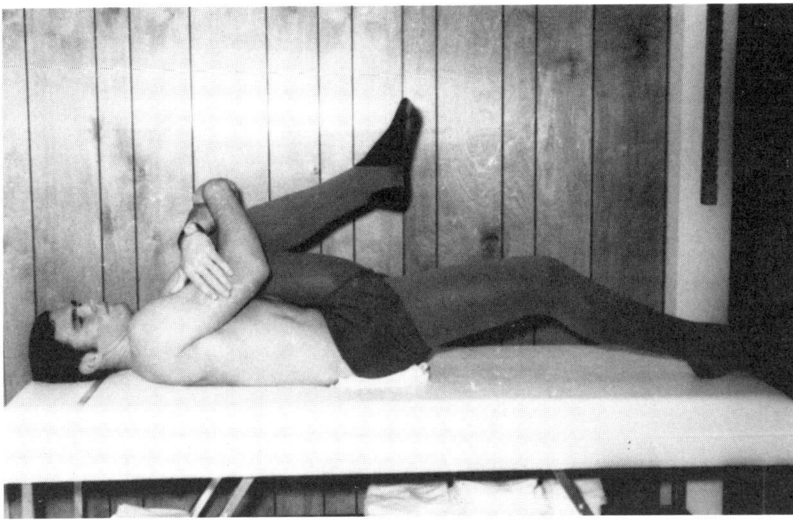

(Shortened Hip Flexors)

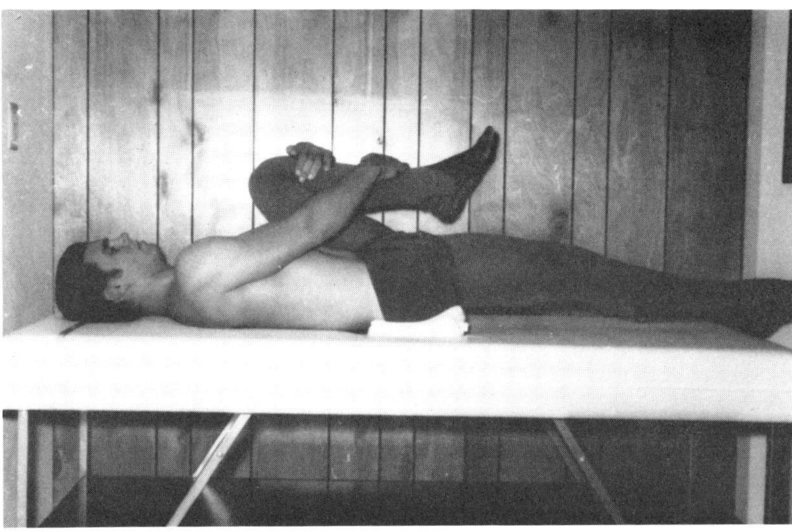

(Lengthened Hip Flexors)

FIGURE 27 Stretching Hip Flexors

If the hip flexors are too short, you continue stretching them gently and frequently until the leg is straight (that is when the thigh is parallel to the low back).

With the low back stretched out and the hip flexors of normal length, you should now be able to stand with your back flat and your legs straight. You should have a feeling of sitting on your legs, without any strain on your low back. If you have to keep your head forward and your shoulders rounded in order to keep your back flat in the standing position, most likely you have an upper back and neck posture problem with shortened muscles in the upper part of your trunk keeping you from straightening out your middle back and neck.

SPINAL CURVES

The spine includes three curves: The cervical or neck curve, the dorsal or mid-back curve, and finally the lumbar or low back curve (figure 28). Now, these three curves are compensatory, that is, the larger one is, the larger the other has to be in order that you may see straight ahead in the standing position. If you are going to lessen one of these curves you must lessen the others proportionately so that you may see straight ahead of you at all times comfortably.

If you want the low back to stay flat, then you must flatten the upper back and neck. If you are unable to straighten the neck and mid-back, you will either be hunched over looking into the ground, or maintaining your neck in a very strained position when you are looking straight ahead.

In order to relieve this neck strain when you are looking forward you would have to lift your rib cage, which would arch your low back and increase the low back curve, causing a strain in the low back and lessening the strain in the neck. We can now conclude that the curves would be exaggerated and in a strained position if any one curve is exaggerated. Consequently, you must be able to flatten out all of the curves of the spine if

FIGURE 28 Spinal Curves

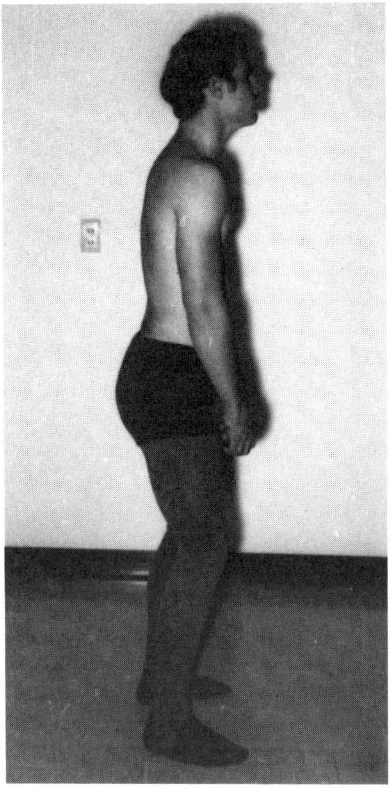

(Exaggerated Curves)

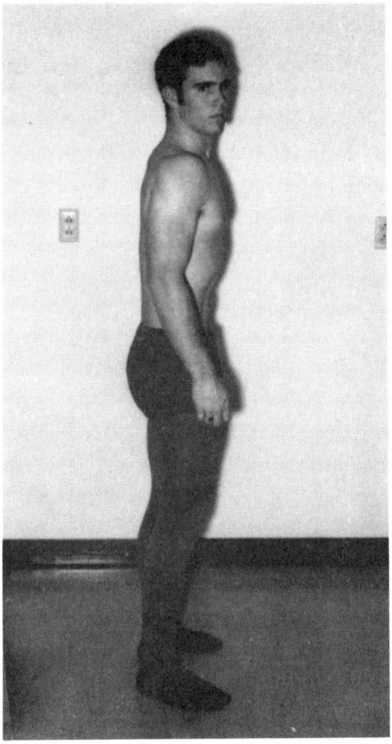

(Lessened or Flattened Spinal Curves)

you want to have the least amount of strain in all the curves and be in the best position to see straight forward when standing.

THE DORSAL CURVE (Mid Back)

The dorsal curve is increased by allowing your shoulders to relax and drop forward, giving the appearance of a sunken chest, round back, and round shoulders (figure 29). This appearance is caused by moving your shoulder joints forward and allowing the lowest portion of your shoulder blades to protrude backwards, creating the appearance of wings. In the process the head is forced forward, which increases the cervical or neck curve. With the increased cervical curve the dorsal curve appears even greater.

When the dorsal curve is maintained in one position for a long period of time, as is done in many older people, the chest muscles called the pectorals and the shoulder extensors, which include many muscles extending from the upper arm backward to the shoulder blade, including a very strong muscle called the latissimus dorsi which extends down to the lower back, become shortened and fix the exaggerated dorsal curve.

STRETCHING SHOULDER EXTENSORS AND PECTORALS

Two exercises are needed to stretch the shortened muscles and other tissue which may be adhesed in order to regain normal flexibility. Without the increased flexibility it is impossible to flatten or lessen these curves.

The starting position for both of these exercises is very similar. Begin by sitting in a chair with your forehead on a table and your arms extended along the side of your head. Keep your head down on the table and raise your arms toward the ceiling, keeping them as close to your ears as possible (figure 30). You should feel a stretching along the outside or lateral aspect of your shoulder joints or the axilla (armpit). As soon as a good stretch is felt, stop and hold the arms up for a count before

FIGURE 29
Rounded Shoulders and Back

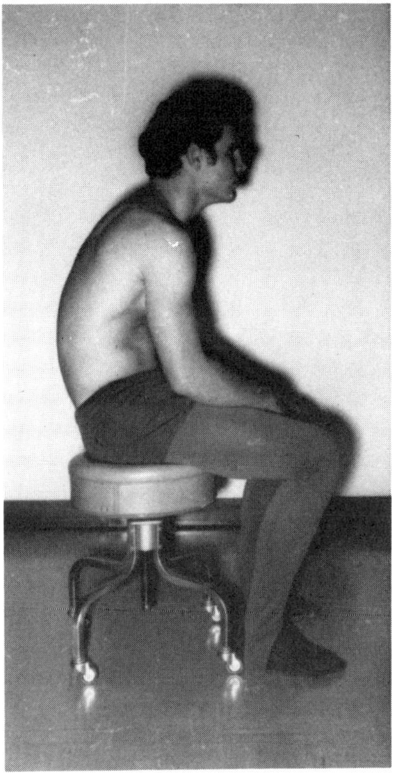

(Exaggerated Dorsal Curve)

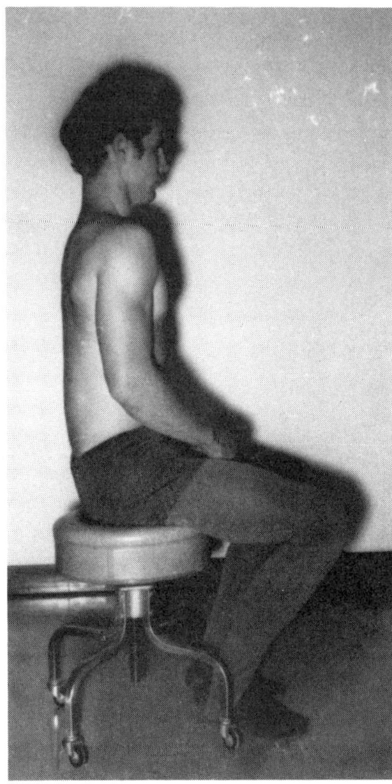

(Straightened Dorsal Curve)

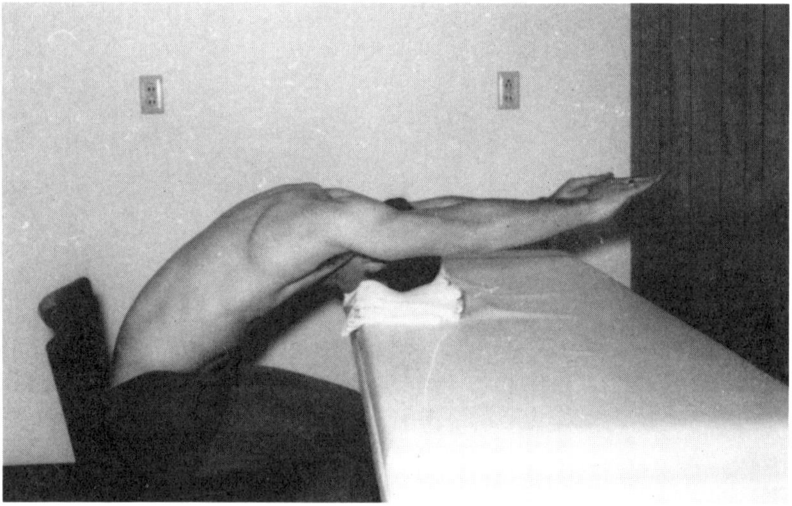

(Shortened Shoulder Extensors)

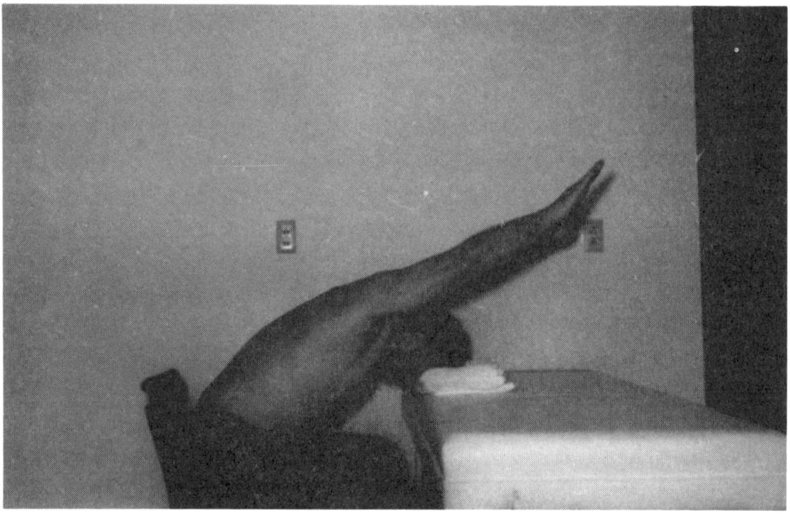

(Stretched Out Shoulder Extensors)

FIGURE 30 Stretching Shoulder Extensors

letting them down. Don't raise them too forcefully or jerkily as you may strain your neck. Relax completely between each stretch; keep your chin in tightly to protect your neck..

To stretch the pectorals or chest muscles, assume the same position with your forehead on the table. Instead of placing your arms outstretched alongside your head, move them out to the side from your head to about forty-five degrees, with your thumbs pointing toward the ceiling. Now slowly raise your arms to the ceiling as far as you can (figure 31). You should feel a stretch in your upper chest muscles, especially nearer your shoulder joints. Hold your arms up for a count in this stretched position before you let them down and relax completely.

When both arms (primarily the elbows) can be raised above the head or to a position even with the top of the head, normal flexibility will be reached. This flexibility should allow you to place your dorsal spine in a flattened position by pulling your shoulder blades back together and down toward your low back.

THE CERVICAL CURVE (Neck)

The cervical curve is very much influenced by the dorsal curve regardless of whether you are sitting or standing. In the standing position all these curves are very much affected equally by each other. However, in the sitting position the lumbar or low back curve is always flattened out.

In the sitting position, if both the dorsal and cervical curves are straight, your head will be looking straight ahead. However, in the standing position they can both be straight and you will not be looking straight ahead if your low back curve is not also straight. Of course, the reason for this is because the low back is always more straight in the sitting position.

It is very difficult to keep the dorsal curve and the cervical curve straight without keeping both straight. For example, if you slouch or relax with your shoulders forward, your head is also forced forward and the cervical or neck curve is greatly increased (figure 29). If you now pull your shoulder blades

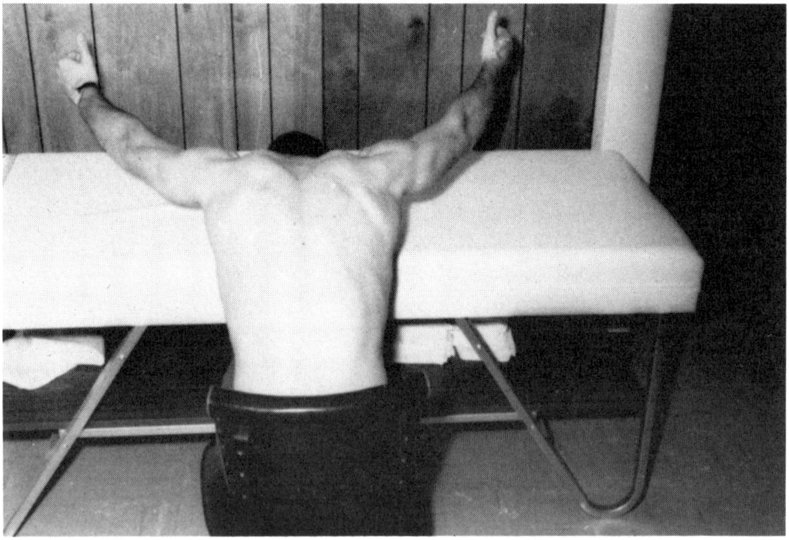

(Shortened Pectoral Muscles)

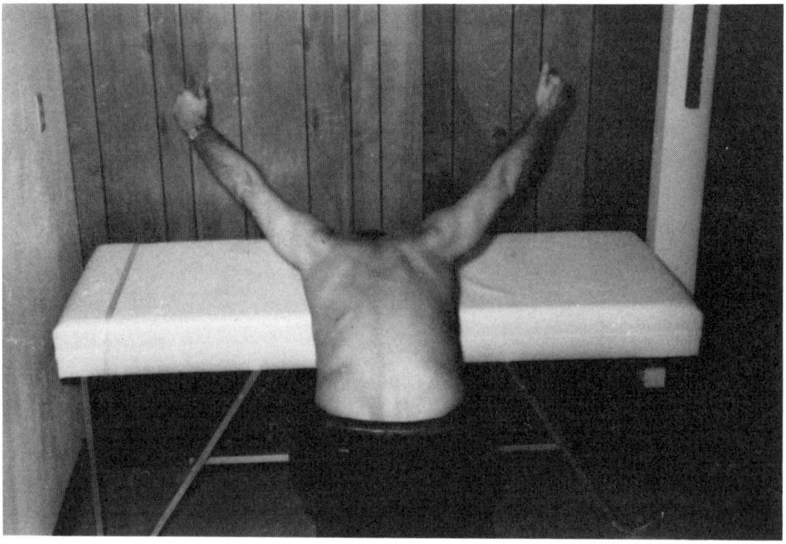

(Lengthened Pectoral Muscles)

FIGURE 31 Stretching Pectorals

back without lifting your chest or rib cage, the head feels very uncomfortable protruding forward and the natural tendency is to bring the head back toward the shoulders. The reverse is true with the head or neck curve. If the neck curve is increased by allowing the head to go forward, the shoulders tend to follow the head, increasing the dorsal curve as the neck curve increases.

The cervical curve becomes fixed by two groups of muscles, the neck extensors which pull your head back as in looking up to the ceiling, and the lateral neck flexors which go from the base of the skull near the ear and extend toward the shoulder joints. These muscles pull your head to the side as when you try touching your ear to your shoulder joint while looking straight ahead.

The neck extensors which pull your head back compare with the string of a bow. The tighter the string the bigger or deeper the bow. The tighter or shorter the neck extensors the deeper or greater is the neck or cervical curve (figure 32). Consequently, these muscles must be long enough so that the cervical curve can be flattened out.

STRETCHING NECK EXTENSORS

The starting position is sitting with the shoulder blades pulled back and down, flattening the dorsal curve as much as possible. In stretching the neck extensors, pull the chin in toward your throat as far as possible and pull your head down toward your chest (figure 33). As you pull your head down, keep pushing your chin in as if to push it up through your throat and into your ears. During this procedure you must forcefully keep your shoulders back and down toward your mid and low back. If this exercise is done properly, the stretching should be felt only in the cervical spine, and considerable pulling may be felt at the base of the skull where the neck extensor muscles insert into the skull. This exercise should be continued until the chin is down on the chest and the head is unable to flex any further. You must be careful not to allow the chin to protrude or slide down the chest when doing this exercise. If you do, you will

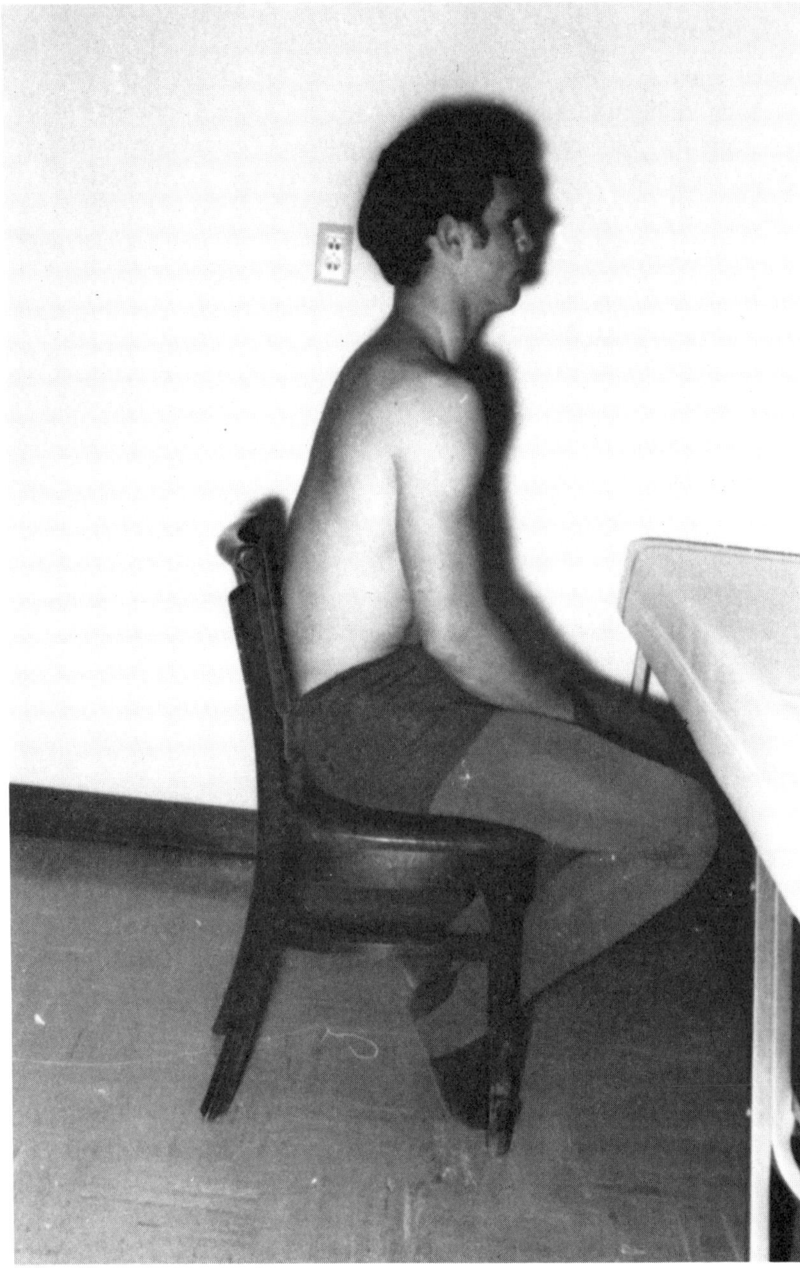

FIGURE 32 Shortened Neck Extensors

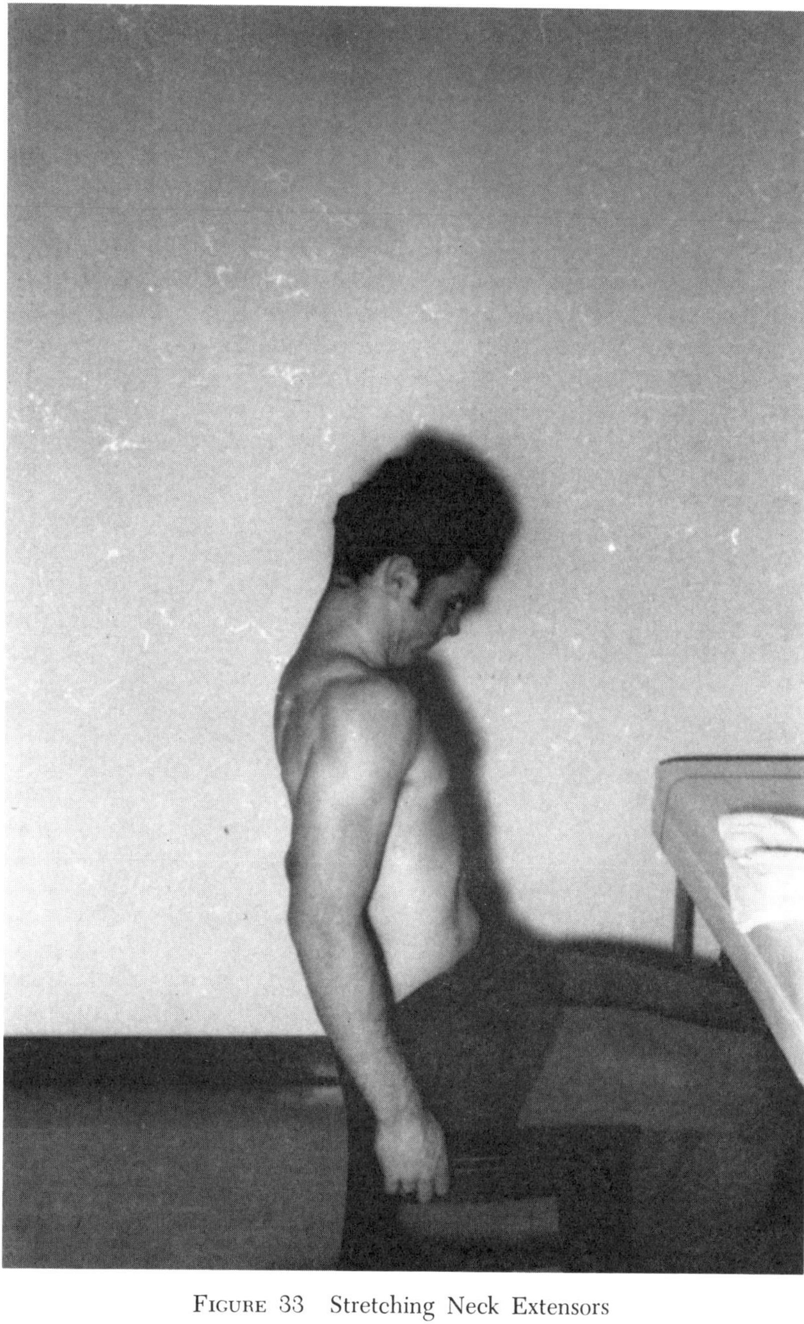

Figure 33 Stretching Neck Extensors

cause a shearing effect in the cervical vertebrae which may produce a strained joint. It would be the same as if you tried to slide your head off your shoulders.

STRETCHING LATERAL NECK FLEXORS

Stretching the lateral neck flexors begins in the sitting position with both dorsal and cervical curves flattened out. Hold on to the seat of the chair that you are sitting on. This will keep you from raising your shoulders. Now, keeping the chin in, bend your head to either side in an attempt to have your ear touch the tip of your shoulder (figure 34). You should feel a pulling along the side of your neck.

STRETCHING HEEL CORDS

The muscles of the back of the calf originate behind the knee and the center of the back of the lower leg. There are two muscles that come together forming a common tendon, and this tendon inserts into the back of the heel. This tendon is called a heel cord.

If these muscles and cord get too short the ankle loses its flexibility, especially when the knee is straight or at 180 degrees. The loss of flexibility is also noted as one squats as to sit on the floor or on one's heels. If they are too short the tendency is to raise up on the toes as you squat. If you don't raise on the toes and keep your heel on the floor, you will fall backwards because of the shortness of the muscles and lack of flexibility. It is impossible to keep your center of gravity over your feet and the heels flat on the floor as you squat down, if the cords are too short (figure 35).

You are probably asking yourself what tight heeel cords would have to do with a strained back. First of all, they may be a factor in causing a back strain. If you have to work in a squatting position and you must maintain your balance only on the balls of your feet, there is a greater chance of injuring your low back because of the poor balance and lack of stability. The

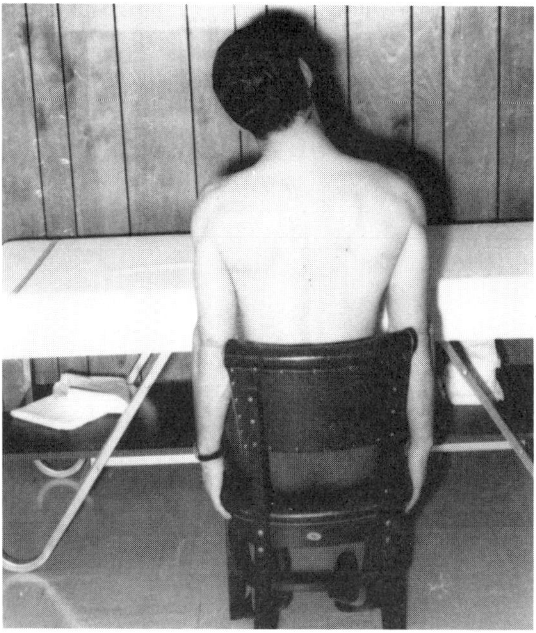

(Shortened Lateral Neck Flexors)

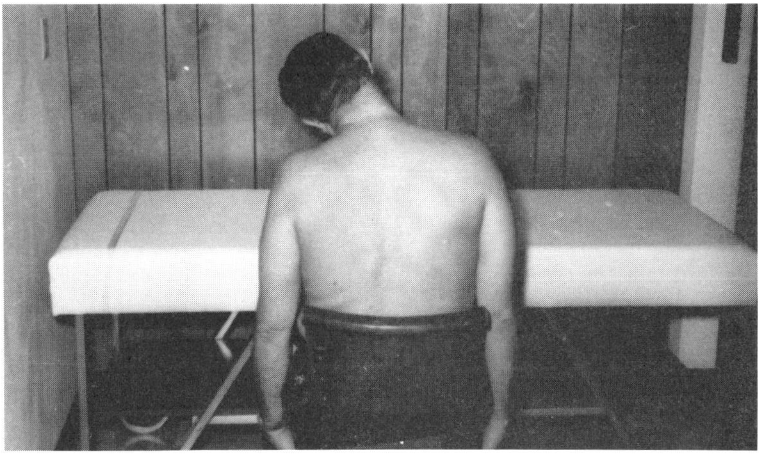

(Lengthened Lateral Neck Flexors)

FIGURE 34 Stretching Lateral Neck Flexors

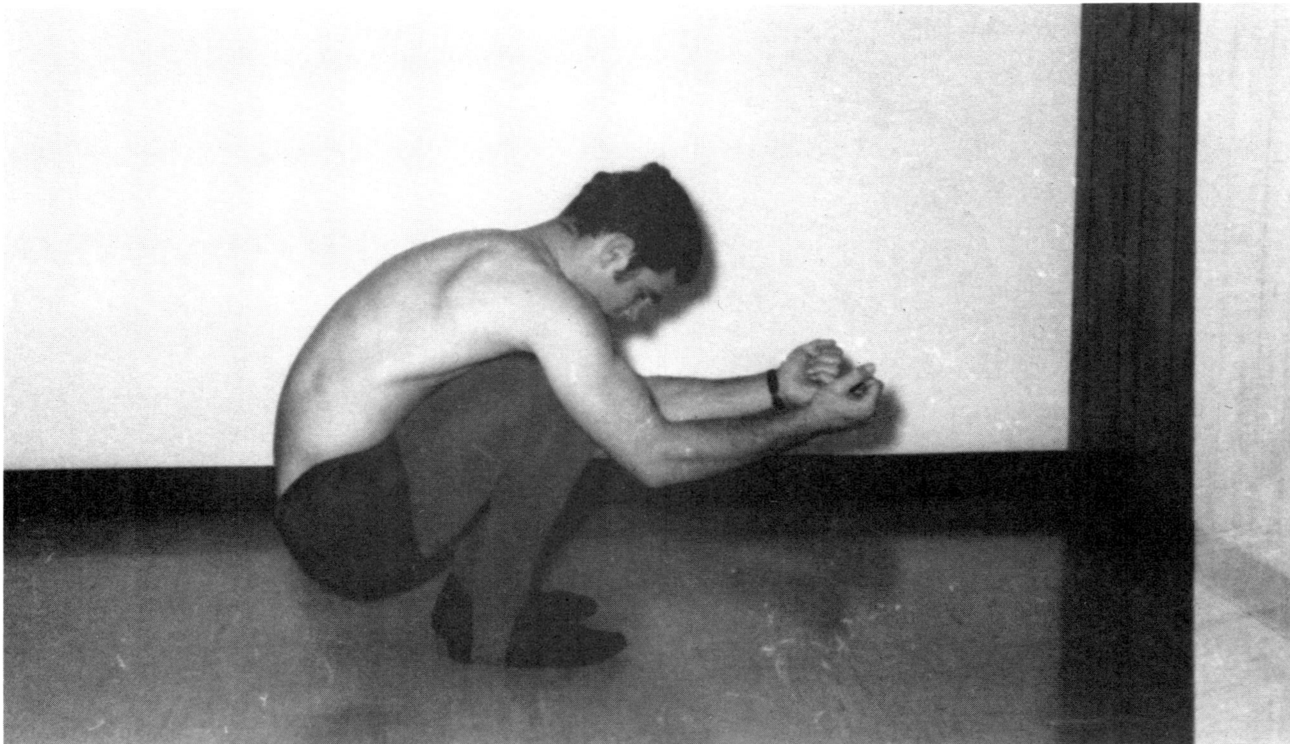

FIGURE 35 Shortened Heel Cords

back is forced into a strained or arched position as you squat in order to keep your balance. As your weight is transferred from the heel to the toes the low back must arch, tilting the rib cage backward to compensate for the weight of the legs and pelvis going forward, and to keep the body from falling on its knees. Consequently, working in this strained position can cause a strained back. Secondly, if one has a strained back, this position can keep a strain from healing by constant irritations and strain.

If the heel cords are of normal length, you are able to squat all the way down and keep your heels on the floor (figure 36). With the heels flat you have excellent balance and you are forced to keep the low back flat and the upper back rounded with the abdominals completely contracted. If you relaxed your abdominals with your feet flat on the floor in a squatting position, you would fall backwards, as your center of gravity would move backwards.

The heel cords can be stretched very simply. Place your hands on a table or wall; then place one leg forward and one leg back as if in a long stride position with both feet perpendicular to the wall and toes pointing straight away. Keep the knee of the back leg locked in 180 degrees. Now move your body toward the wall, keeping the back knee locked and the heel on the floor. As you move forward bend the forward knee allowing your hips to move forward (figure 37). You should feel a stretching feeling extending from the heel cord to the back of the knee. As soon as you feel a good stretch, stop and return to the starting position. After ten repetitions, place the forward leg back, the back leg forward, and stretch as before.

Stretching of heel cords should be done as often as possible during the day until they are long enough to allow you to sit on your heels in the squatting position with your heels flat on the floor. Stretch them gently and frequently.

TECHNIQUES OF EXERCISING

There are other specific exercises which may be of value for back strains. However, I believe they should be done only under the supervision of a doctor or physical therapist.

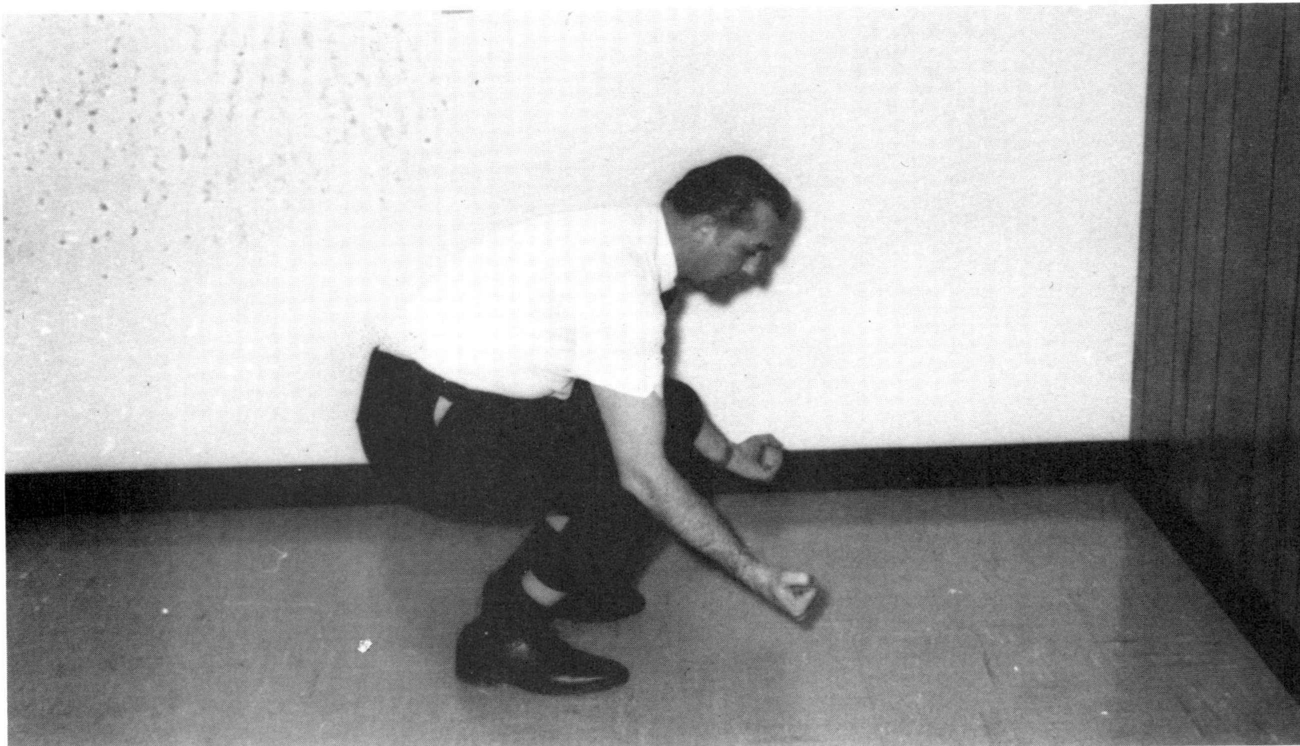

FIGURE 36 Stretched Out Heel Cords

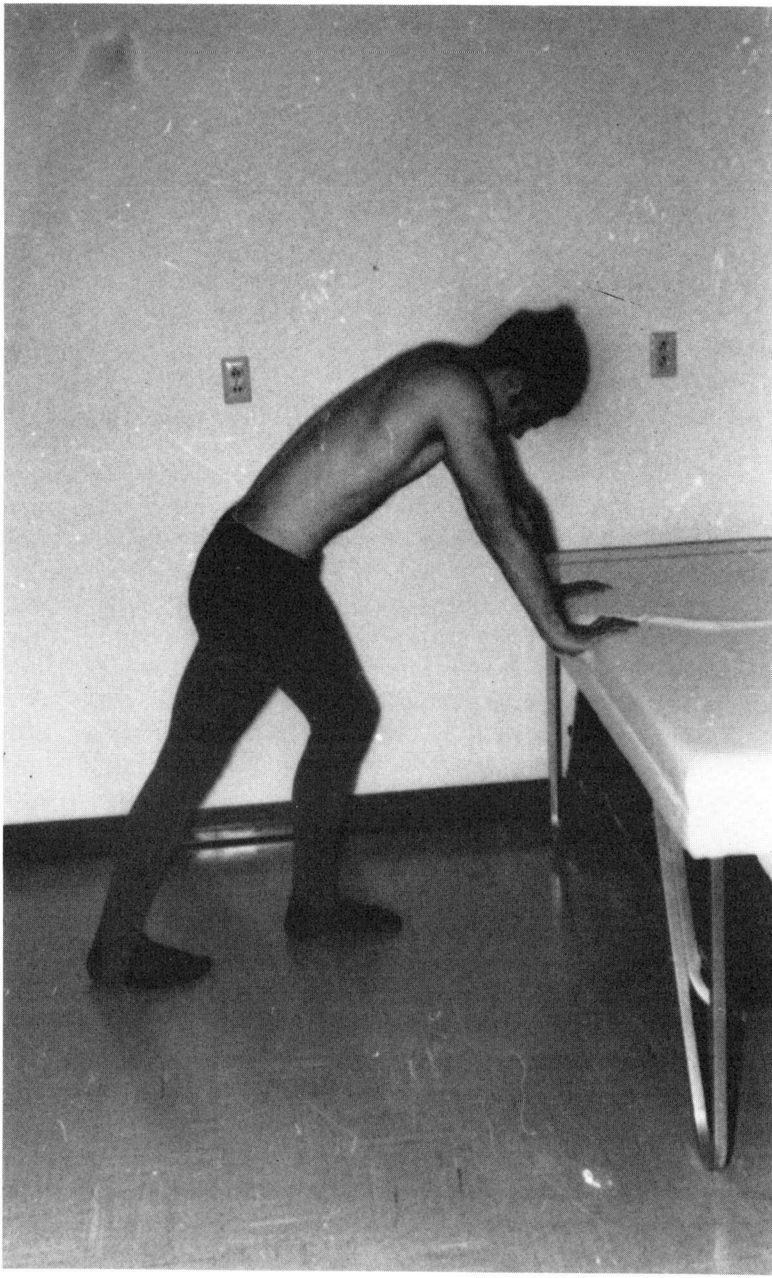

Figure 37 Stretching Heel Cords

The exercises described should be done slowly so that any discomfort or pain can be anticipated. You should stop as soon as you feel a good stretch. At the first sign of pain you must stop. As you become more flexible and less tender, you can be more forceful in your stretching, as long as there is no aggravation of pain or aching. Always rest or relax completely between each repetition. Do not be in a hurry. You will be wiser to do less exercises and do them properly than to do many and irritate yourself by doing them improperly.

If the exercises are done properly, they should be done as often as possible during the day, which may be approximately every two hours. You should imagine that you are stretching rubber bands. If you stretch them gently and frequently, they will become longer and longer. If you stretch them too forcefully they may tear or break, or the bones may take abnormal positions and cause pain.

You can safely start doing each exercise four or five times every two hours. Each day add one or two repetitions until you are doing each exercise fifteen times every two hours. If severe discomfort is produced, you must stop the exercises temporarily. If the discomfort subsides, that means that you were either doing your exercises too forcefully or too often. Consequently, you should do them more gently and not as often. Everyone should decide for himself as to the force and frequency, as no two people are alike and will be affected differently. It is wiser to start very gently and gradually increase the force and frequency.

If pain is increased and there is no progress when you do your exercises gently, you should consult your doctor. You may have a more serious back problem than a strain.

Exercises should be continued frequently until the normal range of motion is reached and all pain has discontinued. Once the range of motion is normal, further stretching or forcing must not be done as it is possible to strain other joints such as the hip and shoulder joints. Overstretching with exercises is dangerous, as it creates instability. However, the exercises should be continued to maintain the normal range of motion without forcing and trying to increase further motion. The exercises will maintain normal motion while the injured or weakened tissue is healing.

When pain has cleared up completely, you may cut the exercises down to once a day for a month; then three times a week for another month; then twice a week for a month. In three months the injured tissue should be healed and your proper habits with constant use of your abdominals should be established. Then you can discontinue your exercises as there would be no need for them; you will be doing them all day long when you function properly.

EXERCISES AND FUNCTIONAL TRAINING

By this time you should be well aware of the difference and the values of exercise and functional training.

The actual treating of the back is the functional training which is based on contracting and maintaining the abdominal muscles in a complete contraction, preventing movement in the injured joint.

The exercises are to increase flexibility and range of motion so that the abdominal muscles may contract more easily and forcefully and allow the bones to be placed in a strain-free position.

What you do all day long and how you do it is much more significant than how many and what kind of exercises you do. If you are going to eliminate one, eliminate the exercises, since by doing everything properly you will eventually increase your flexibility and strength, although it will take you a longer period of time. It is not so important what you do but what is happening to your back while you are doing it.

Chapter VIII

BRACES, EXERCISE, AND FUNCTIONAL TRAINING

The purpose of all back braces is to prevent movement in the low back, especially in the injured joints. If you used your abdominal muscles as described you would be accomplishing this purpose and a back brace would be unnecessary.

It is impossible for most back braces to prevent all movement in an injured joint in the low back. This can only be done with your abdominal muscles. This is so because the tension is proportional to the pressure on your abdomen. Since the pressures in the abdomen change with breathing, the amount of bulk in your intestines, and the pressure that you can be comfortable with, the tension supporting your low back changes accordingly. Also, the brace is attached firmly to the top of the pelvis. Regardless of how tight the brace is fastened, the lower portion of the pelvis and the sacrum can still be tipped backward, arching the low back. It is also impossible to keep the rib cage from raising with the brace for the same reason. There is constant movement inside a brace unless the abdominal muscles are contracted firmly as described throughout this book. The brace does prevent excess movement and this may be of considerable value to many people who have a mild weakness and have discomfort only in the extreme range of extension or arching of the back.

Braces are usually fitted in a normal standing position to fit your individually curved spine. If you have a deep arch or sway, the brace is adjusted to fit the curve and maintain the curve, regardless of how deep it is. It doesn't make much sense to brace an injured joint in a strained position. When you sit down, the same curve must be maintained in the sitting position; otherwise, if you relax, you will experience pain in the center of the curve. Since the low back normally flattens out in the sitting position and the brace keeps you from flattening your back, you are most uncomfortable.

The sad part of this type of bracing, which is being done everywhere, is that it prevents healing by keeping the joints of the low back in an unfavorable position during all activity.

Braces should be fitted in a perfect sitting position. The pelvis should be perpendicular to the seat and the low back flat. The rib cage should be directly over the pelvis with the sternum perpendicular to the seat. In this position the center of gravity from the low back up should be directly through the injured joint or anterior to it. The brace should be high enough in front to keep the rib cage from tilting backward.

If you are braced properly the low back should be in the same position in the standing position as it was in the sitting position. It should also be maintained in the same position during all activities. However, as I said before, it is impossible to prevent movement in a brace except with your abdominal muscles, which you should learn to use if you must wear a brace.

If you find it difficult to keep your back flat in the brace in the standing position, most likely your hip flexors are shortened and should be stretched as explained in the section on therapeutic exercise. The needed flexibility will allow you to flatten the back and fit the brace as you are fitted in the sitting position.

Strengthening the abdominals is a must when wearing a brace, as there is a tendency to depend on the brace to do the work of the abdominals. Over a long period of time the abdominals may become very weak if not exercised or used properly inside the brace. The brace should never be discarded unless the abdominal muscles are strong enough and trained well enough to support the low back.

Remember that if you must wear a brace it should be fitted to you while your back is in the most favorable strain-free position. This can only be when the back is flattened out as it is when the abdominals are contracted completely. This may be very uncomfortable at first, but you must learn to work with the brace fitted properly and your back in the pain-free position.

Bracing should be done only when necessary, as it is a crutch replacing the abdominal muscles. If you must wear a brace you should learn all the basic movements as described in this book and use your abdominal muscles constantly, since it is impossible to keep the joint absolutely quiet in a brace even if you are braced properly. By doing this you will not be afraid to remove the brace. There are many situations, such as moving in bed, taking a bath or shower, or partaking in intercourse, when the brace must be removed. By learning to use your abdominal muscles properly, there is much less chance of irritating or re-injuring the joint when the brace is removed.

Chapter IX

PREVENTION

PREVENTION OF LOW BACK STRAIN

Since back strain is a national and international problem, it should be attacked on a national and international plane. As mentioned earlier, millions of dollars are being spent to treat and prevent back strain. Millions of dollars more are lost in inefficiency and lack of production in industry because of back pain. The misery and pain the people experience because of back pain is immeasurable.

In order to make any significant impact on back problems we must eliminate the causes. The causes are lack of flexibility, lack of abdominal muscle strength, and the improper use of the abdominal muscles and the spine. To eliminate causes, people must be informed as to what they are and they must act upon them. One without the other will produce failure, as everyone must be motivated to act by knowledge. Once they are informed and motivated, situations must be created in which this knowledge can be put into practice.

PREVENTION IN SCHOOL AND HOME

The first step in informing and motivating must take place in our school system, beginning with the first grade and extending through all the grades. In order to inform and motivate all the students, the teachers must first be informed and motivated. Parents can also be informed and motivated through part of the educational system such as the PTA. They should then act and set examples.

Teachers, especially physical education teachers, can administer exercises for flexibility and strength. All teachers should feel a responsibility to teach good posture, functional training, and the proper use of the abdominal muscles. The spine is affected by all activities of daily living, as explained in this book. Consequently, how students stand, sit, get up or sit down in classrooms can be of utmost importance. If a teacher is indifferent, so will her or his students be.

As students become older and new activities such as dancing, gymnastics, and athletics become a part of their curriculum, they should be taught how to participate with maximum flexibility and proper use of the abdominal muscles.

The need for teaching and the methods will vary from age group to age group. During the early teen years there is marked growth and change in appearance, weight, and attitudes. Students become much more self-conscious. These are the years during which the most effort should be put forth to maintain flexibility, proper posture, and functional training.

During the elementary school years, flexibility should be stressed. Possibly 50 percent of all young school children have shortened hip flexors because of their swaybacked posture which results from parents' attitudes and the hereditary structure of muscle and bones. Normal flexibility of the hips and shoulders can be regained and maintained by proper exercises while proper posture and function are being taught.

Preschool children can be taught by their parents. Parents can be taught through the PTA, churches, services organizations, and industry.

For those students that continue on with higher education, a constructive program should be carried on in all colleges and universities. Here again all teachers, especially physical education teachers, should be trained in proper use of the abdominal muscles in posture and functional training. Exercise programs should be required of all students to maintain or regain their necessary flexibility during their years of study.

Once a successful program is established at home and in school, it must be continued and followed through in industry and all forms of employment.

PREVENTION IN INDUSTRY

Industry should be most concerned about preventing back strain, as it is carrying the financial burden of paying most of the medical treatment. Health and accident premiums continue to skyrocket because of increased paid benefits resulting from inflation, increased injuries, and increased benefits. The increased benefits are primarily due to increased injuries. In most injury cases, industry must pay compensation to the workers while they are not working. These benefits may be even greater than the cost of medical treatment. The financial losses in industry because of injuries are staggering. The unmeasurable loss of production is probably equally staggering.

How many people today are working with back pain from mild to severe degrees? How many of these people are able to work at normal to maximum efficiency? How are these people affecting the efficiency and production of workers who do not have back pain? How much total production is being lost? The answers to these questions would be most revealing.

All people who have back pain or any other pain have a fear of their pain becoming worse; consequently, they move and act defensively. They move deliberately, for fear of making a mistake and aggravating their condition. Their speed, coordination, and reaction time are seriously slowed down. Favoring of the back because of pain results in incoordination and lack of strength. With the lack of speed, reaction time, coordination, and strength, efficiency and production are lost.

When people cannot function normally and efficiently, they

are susceptible to further injury. They may also be the cause of other people getting injured. For example, let us consider two people carrying a heavy object down the stairs, one of whom has a back problem. If the person with the back pain must let go suddenly, the normal person could injure his back with the excess strain. Other injuries such as a hernia or a broken foot bone may result. A person with a weak back may expect a normal person to carry more of a load, resulting in an injury. A truck driver with a back pain may not be able to step on the brake as fast as he normally would. The result could be a serious accident. The consequences of such an accident may include additional injuries to the driver, injuries to other people, material losses including the truck, loss of time, effects on production, and finally the cost of settling such a problem.

An industry can decrease the problem of back strain and related injuries by changing the worker and changing his environment.

Workers should regain the lost flexibility of the shoulders, hips, and ankles. This is best done by proper exercises, as explained thoroughly in the chapter on therapeutic exercise. This can be accomplished also with pamphlets, pictures, demonstrations and ten-minute exercise periods during the day and at home. Each worker could be evaluated and taught only the exercises that he needs. This situation, of course, would be ideal.

Increased flexibility will prevent many other injuries. People who are flexible very rarely injure themselves by falling, as is demonstrated by the falls of young children and tumblers. This is so because of the give and the lack of rigidity when a blow is applied. Increased flexibility will increase coordination which will improve job performance and prevent injury by improving body control and balance. Increased flexibility will improve posture, which will result in improved appearance, improved circulation, reduced fatigue, and the improved mental attitude of the worker. This, in turn, will improve the mental attitudes of his fellow workers.

Once flexibility is regained, everyone must be taught how to use his abdominal muscles properly, as shown in this book. Even if normal flexibility is not regained, proper use of the abdominals should be taught. This is the only manner in which back strain can be prevented and cured.

If industry expects the workers to do their part by regaining their flexibility and learning how to use their abdominal muscles properly, industry must do its part in helping to prevent back injury.

Industry's responsibility is to give the worker the opportunity to do his part, and to arrange the capital or environment in the most favorable position in which it can produce the most goods with the least chance of injury. For example, the heights of work tables should be questioned. They should be determined by the job being done and the size of the workman. If the work is minute and difficult to see, the tables should be higher and closer to the head of the workman. If a job requires a great deal of straining, the height of the table should correspond to the best and most efficient position for the worker to strain in. In many situations, it may be wiser to raise the position of the worker than the work table or machine. It may be also, in many situations, more advantageous and more efficient to move people rather than parts and equipment.

Production and accidents are strongly influenced by attitudes. Workers who are in pain, or have fear of becoming worse, or have a fear of becoming injured, are sad and depressing to themselves and to their fellow workers. They cannot function with confidence. Their ability to concentrate on their specific job or responsibility is limited, resulting in poor production and negative thinking. Such negative attitudes are contagious and influence normal happy people negatively. The positive, cheerful, clear-thinking worker enjoys solving problems, and produces and radiates enthusiasm for his work and for other people.

Teaching workers how to condition their bodies properly and how to function efficiently without pain is most important in changing attitudes and establishing self-confidence. Workers who are physically and mentally normal or better conditioned will produce most efficiently.

There are as many ways for industry to prevent back strain as there are creative people who can understand the mechanical problems of the human body as well as the mechanical problems of industry.

Chapter X

SUMMARY AND CONCLUSION

SUMMARY

I have taken the basic movements of the body such as standing, sitting, walking, getting up and down from a squatting or a sitting position, and twisting and reaching, and discussed how the abdominal muscles control movement in the low back to prevent pain. I further discussed how these basic movements are involved in all activities of daily living such as lifting, pushing, climbing, running, ascending, descending, working, recreation, sports, and even pregnancy and intercourse.

Exercises were taught to increase flexibility of the entire spine, hips, shoulders, and ankles, in order to place all the bones in the most advantageous positions for allowing the abdominals to work more efficiently and forcefully when necessary.

Finally, I presented a plan for prevention which would involve our educational system, our industries, service organizations, churches, and, most of all, each individual.

CONCLUSION

I would like to conclude with a hope that I have accomplished what I intended to do, which was to teach anyone with a back strain or sprain how to function without pain, by knowing how to use the abdominal muscles properly, and also to show how one may keep from getting a back strain.

I truly believe, after teaching and treating low back strains for nineteen years in this manner, that anyone who sincerely follows this program will cure himself permanently and will be able to happily say, "There Goes My Aching Back."